I0830495

For Love's Sake

A guide to improving you, your relationships, and the world
we share.

By Leonard F. Schwank

Copyright © 2021 Leonard F. Schwank

All rights reserved. No part of this book may be reproduced or used in any manner without written permission of the copyright owner except for the use of quotations used or within a book review. Please share this book with your friends and family in an attempt to share the love and improve their relationships.

Thank you for your support, enjoy!

Love is like a flower that will grow into its full potential given water, sunlight, and a healthy foundation. These few necessities are similar to the relatively simple yet often misunderstood foundations for a healthy relationship. Through a series of heartbreaks and failures, I began to discover and understand these principles. By sharing my experiences and mistakes, I hope to ease your struggles in love and increase your chances of success. I'll provide you with insight and real life examples of how to find, maintain, and make the most of your ever-evolving love situation.

If you're ready for a lasting and meaningful overhaul of your love life, this book is for you. I want you to find the excitement, hope, and comfort that love can provide. The kind of love that gives you a reason to get up in the morning and leaves you with a smile on your face at the end of the day. No matter if you're new to the dating game or have been married so long that dementia has turned the years into a love-less slurry, your love life **will** improve if you take these pages to heart and apply them to your life. Love is a powerful force and I hope to help you put that power to work. If I can inspire even one person to practice love more successfully, I will consider these pages worth the effort.

I've seen many romance movies, and if you stop to think about the progression of each of these stories, there is a common theme. **Passion**. The characters are willing to risk life and limb for the sake of their future love. All of their toils in the name of love are in pursuit of the seemingly elusive *happy-ending*. These happy-endings are earned through dedication, conscious effort, and a blind hope for the future. If you were to utilize these romance movies scenarios as the blueprint for a relationship, I'd be willing to bet that the relationship would end just as quickly as it began. Oftentimes, your happy ending will turn out significantly less *magical*, and the romance you were hoping for may not come in the package you were expecting. The problem with these movies is that we only see the *happy-ending* and are left to speculate on how the rest of their romantic lives play out. What happens a month after their exciting honeymoon? They're probably fighting over mundane things and minor aspects of daily life. Instead of living an idealistic fantasy about how love should be, understand that to correctly lay or fix a relationship foundation, there will be times when you want to quit and might wonder- where is my *happy-ending*. If you put in the work, it will come. Maybe not as you were expecting, but that's what makes love so exciting. I'll take a complicated and exciting relationship that has weathered many trials and tribulations over a shallow love any day.

I'll teach you how to reach that happy ending without any of the desperation or other hang-ups that many romance movies idealize. Unlike love at first sight and the few minor hiccups presented throughout romance movies, it actually takes hard work to continuously grow in a relationship.

These movies create subconscious beliefs that love just happens easily without getting into the nuts-and-bolts of the daily effort required for success. By understanding some of the fundamental principles that can make or break your relationship, you'll be a step-ahead in your love-life. There's no easy solution to the wild problems you'll face in the world of love, but if you have a big heart, courage, and a solid work-ethic, you'll end up with the kind of love you deserve. I don't care what your definition of love is, but if you're completely honest with yourself, you already know that you need it. We all do. And regardless of the vision you have for your love life, just like any worthy goal, it takes effort to improve and grow. By learning how to cater to your loved ones with a new attitude and perspective, your life will exponentially unfold in ways you never thought possible. But don't take my word for it. Come back to this book a year from now and reflect on just how much you've grown in your relationship.

Of course, conditions apply - **you have to be willing to work for love** if you hope to achieve a love that is worth fighting for. Without worthy sacrifice, there is no worthy reward. When you feel like your wheels are spinning in any of the areas we cover, don't let doubt creep in and discourage you. If challenging situations didn't knock you down from time to time, you would never become resilient. Adapt to your circumstances by learning to forgive yourself and analyze why things didn't work out like you had hoped. The ideas I present to you are simply that, ideas. You might not agree with the solutions I present to you, but hopefully they will encourage you to think about your situation from a different perspective. When you find that a solution isn't working out as planned, change course and keep trying to approach the problem with a new strategy. The strongest relationships are the ones that figured out the solutions rather than giving up when times were tough.

I'm a self-proclaimed lover (or fighter when fighting for love) and have done some seriously insane and stupid things for the sake of finding, holding onto, or escaping from love.

Maybe you aren't even looking for love or a relationship in the traditional sense. We each have different ideas of what our love life should include, and perhaps, you already know that you prefer the single life. This book is still relevant to you. All of the ideas presented in this book are designed to help you grow in **every** kind of relationship.

Just the idea of love is enough to make an otherwise sane and well-balanced individual transform into a ravenous beast that has lost all connection with reality. That's why countless songs, books, and movies have been made on the subject; all attempting (mostly in vain) to demystify the subtlety and wonder of its inner-workings. Love is a complex issue. Don't be discouraged if you haven't quite figured it out yet. If finding and maintaining a quality love life was simple, you'd miss out on the depth and beauty that comes from a relationship that has made it through hell and back. Despite the complexity of love, and the high-probability that you'll never master the craft, the important thing is to continue learning and growing.

The truth is, love can and probably will hurt you. The staggering number of broken relationships across the world is testament to the seemingly inescapable reality that truly successful relationships take dedicated work and conscious effort. Do you have the desire to have a fulfilling relationship that is both challenging yet equally rewarding? Then you'll need to have an equal level of resolve in order to take the steps necessary to succeed. I hope you're ready to fight for love.

The reality of "love"

In order to cultivate the love life you're hoping for, it's important to understand some of the genetic predispositions that often lead us to failure. We are hard-wired to survive. Unfortunately for our romantic lives, survival and long-term commitment are at odds. Our ancestors were only concerned with the necessities: food, water, shelter, and surviving just long enough to reproduce and keep the blood-line flowing.

Unlike our ancestors, our modern desire for commitment and romantic love is a by-product of the relative ease of survival today. When you look back into human history, you'll find that romantic love was not necessary. A committed relationship had little realistic value. Instead, sharing multiple partners led to diverse blood-lines with many alternative genetic dispositions. Now that our basic needs are met with modern agriculture and access to necessary supplies, we are pioneers in this new era of love. We are enabled to explore and enjoy things that our ancestors could only dream of. While they might have been concerned over the success of their next hunt, we are concerned over the amount of likes we get on our Facebook feed.

Understanding the origins of our success as a human species is imperative to mastering love in the modern world. Against all of our instinctual drivers, we must consciously choose to accept the new paradigm of love that is available to us. Instead of viewing our natural tendency to want a new or different partner as inherently wrong, we can view these urges from a higher perspective. With the knowledge that you aren't *wrong* for desiring a new partner, you can acknowledge these feelings without reacting instinctually and continuously remain loyal to your current partner. That's entirely up to you. Perhaps you are destined to continue hopping from partner to partner. But if you prefer the committed life, you'll be more resilient with the knowledge that at the end of the day, we are wired to survive, rather than pursue endless romance.

When tempted by the fruit of another, you can choose to continue loving your current partner rather than caving to primal desires. On a genetic level there is a battle being waged against your senses; your body wants constant diversity and to reproduce endlessly, but on a love level, you know that dedication can lead to great fulfillment in life. You don't need multiple partners to keep humanity alive, but you do need to consciously choose loyalty if you want to have a committed relationship.

Another important reality of love to consider is the annoyance factor. At the beginning of any relationship, you might find yourself smiling and swooning over every little detail. You love the way they laugh, the way they smell, and every other little thing about them. Unfortunately, those same nuances are likely to morph into the very things you despise down the road. The hard truth is that your partner will annoy you. Unless you're living in denial, it's probably pretty easy to pick a few things about your past or current partner that rub you the wrong way.

Once again, we need to reflect back on instinctual survival. We are designed to be on constant alert for the next life-ending threat. Our minds are quick to notice the flaws and errors in our immediate surroundings. Unfortunately, this reflects in our astounding ability to hyper-focus on the perceived flaws in our partners. The aspects of our relationships that involve love, kindness, and support are often taken for granted subconsciously because these examples don't represent immediate threats. It means your brain is functioning properly; the need to survive was a priority in the past. But, perhaps the tables have turned and you're hoping to unlearn your ancestors' established defense mechanisms. In order to combat the *perceived flaw bias* that can easily arise in a relationship, practicing a more conscious and appreciative approach to love is a powerful solution.

Our modern love paradigm doesn't mesh well with this outdated protection mechanism. By understanding this natural propensity to seek out the dangers in life, we can become conscious of the deception our minds create. The next time you feel irritated by someone or something, reflect on your primal wiring and remind yourself that your brain is in defense mode. Is the person really doing something that horrible, or is your mind just focused on the problem? It's not your fault. Blame your ancestors.

Instead of letting our pre-programming run the show, it's time to become more conscious of the way we perceive our partners. We can do this a number of ways with nothing other than a simple shift in what we choose to focus on. Every time you feel a frustration arise, I challenge you to combat these occurrences with an internal counter-point. Are you upset that there is a dirty dish in the sink? Well, maybe they folded your laundry yesterday. Are you upset because they forgot to send that Christmas card to your parents? Well, look at the 300$ smart watch on your wrist that they worked so hard for. When we consciously choose to remember the positive experiences in our relationship, the perceived issues lose their all-powerful status.

The concept of unlearning our primal software is closely tied to the gradual shift to a more appreciative outlook in life. Later in this book, I'll detail some techniques for establishing a more solution-oriented and appreciative mindset that will make unlearning our defensive states a realistic objective. I will show you how you can begin taking steps today that will change the way you see yourself and your love life. Are you willing to take the often uncomfortable and treacherous path to lasting change?

Learning to let go of attachment in love and life

I have learned many hard lessons throughout my relationship journey. From a young age, I've always been curious and constantly questioned why things worked the way they do. As my understanding and grasp of the world around me grew, so did my self-confidence. This led to courage and an outspoken nature that naturally attracted the opposite sex. Up until then, I thought I had the world figured out, so figuring out girls would be simple right?

Goodness was I wrong. Girls are complicated. I was addicted to the chase; the adrenaline filled experience of coming clean to a crush and finding out that they felt the same. The blind excitement and optimism for a future together without a care in the world.

It all seemed so wonderful.
Until it wasn't.
Time and time and time again.

I thought to myself, "How unlucky am I? I just keep striking out. I'm doing everything right but these girls are impossible!"

Through a series of painful heartbreaks and tear-filled endings, I began to learn an important lesson about humility. Fortunately for me, this lesson didn't come easily. I didn't realize at the time that all of the misery I was experiencing was the best relationship coach one could ask for. While my confidence and kind attitude would get me in the door, those attributes were not enough to sustain the relationships. I was discovering that while success in school or work could be reached through calculated planning, this was not the case for relationships. The turbulent and inevitable failures that I faced while serial dating motivated me to reflect on what was at the core of these failures. Having a multitude of previously failed relationships gave me the insight and a large enough sample pool to justify my newly discovered relationship hypothesis: My selfish attitude was a primary cause of the relationship failures.

As I began to hold myself accountable, my perspective from a selfish mindset into one of graciousness slowly emerged. This progress made all of the difference. This mindset shift wasn't immediate, so of course there were growing pains along the way, but gradually this transition into a more consistently giving and caring mentality resulted in nothing short of a miracle. I found a renewed sense of hope as my failures became less pronounced and my relationships lasted longer. I want you to experience this shift. Once you understand that your partner isn't there to serve you, you too will find renewed hope in your love life. It's time to get out of your own way. You might be the problem, but not for long.

Along with the mindset shift towards a more giving attitude, I began studying various philosophical paradigms that are less conventional in American society. Buddhist, Zen, and Stoic philosophers resonated with my world-view, and I began to unlearn the behaviors of our societies' materialistic and vain- centric programming. I'm not going to go into too much detail about my spiritual beliefs, but I encourage you to do some research into non-traditional belief systems to explore for yourself. Acquiring additional knowledge from alternate sources broadens your world view. Anything you can do to expand your understanding of what it takes to create a well-rounded and contented life will benefit your relationship.

One of the most love-relevant principles found in all religious texts is the concept of tithing. This concept is intertwined with the principle of freedom from attachment. Give of yourself freely (stop clinging to your stuff and those around you) and you will have abundance in life. This includes everything from consumer goods to the way you have been dealing with your relationship. Learning to become an amazing lover requires that you slowly learn to let go of hindering attachments. This includes any ideas you might have about your relationship that are centered in superficial desires or false expectations.

Giving of yourself is the perfect catalyst for beginning to unwind from the web of attachment. When we learn that the things we cling to are simply chains holding us back from our true potential, you'll find that creating a cohesive bond with your loved one is much simpler.

Start with some simple changes. Perhaps you're addicted to online shopping. Are you about to buy another pair of shoes that will collect dust in the closet? Have you considered spending that money on a romantic evening with your partner instead?

Attachment within a relationship can be difficult to identify. You may perceive your role within the partnership as an independent entity. While a relationship may be possible with two independent personalities, ultimately long term success requires that we allow ourselves to become vulnerable. By allowing ourselves to ask for help, reveal our weaknesses, and share our true selves with our partners, we are on a path towards undoing the rigid stance of independence. We are not islands. By learning to become vulnerable, we are also undoing the deception of attachment to self that we call independence. When we humble ourselves and acknowledge that we need a partner that supports, encourages, and enables our growth, we are one step closer to freedom from the attachment that defines most failed relationships.

The attachment evident in many relationships comes in many different forms. A few prominent examples ranging from selfish attachment to co-dependence include: overwhelming feelings of loneliness when separated, resentment related to expectations not being met, or unrealistic expectations of the need to be included in all aspects of their life. While seemingly unrelated and at opposite ends of the attachment spectrum, both selfish attachment and co-dependence are in the same boat.

Unlearning limiting attachment behaviors will have profound benefits in your love life. To illustrate this point, let's break-down a situation that might arise within a co-dependent relationship.

Johnny is an introvert that prefers staying at home. Rachel is a party-animal that loves adventuring around town. Despite their glaring introverted/extroverted differences, they have found comfort in each other's company. They have magical chemistry and always finish each other's sentences. They do everything together and are attached at the hip. When they are separated, they feel like something is missing and have come to rely on each other to avoid the pain of loneliness.

As time goes on, Rachel begins to develop resentment for Johnny because he always wants to sit around at home. Rachel feels obligated to stay home with Johnny because of his introverted nature but fails to express her adventurous needs while trying to appease his desires. She loves Johnny and wants to do whatever it takes to make him happy, even at the expense of her own.

In this example, the co-dependence between Rachel and Johnny eventually leads to resentment. Instead of following her heart, Rachel gives up on her true passions in life out of fear that Johnny will leave. By remaining attached to the idea that she has to live her life on his introverted terms rather than expressing her outgoing desires, relationship damage is guaranteed. If Rachel had taken action to remain true to herself, it's likely that Johnny would still have just as much love for her (if not more) rather than feeling like he was left behind. As an introvert, he might actually appreciate some time alone. The end result if there was less attachment? Rachel would have less resentment, and Johnny would learn to appreciate their less frequent time together even more.

While there are countless examples of attachment within relationships, it would be difficult to pin-point an example that benefits a relationship. Less attachment doesn't mean less love, rather, it's the opposite. When we let go of our expectations of how that person should fit in with our world-view, we can fully enjoy the person for their unique qualities rather than judging them for what they aren't. No person can live up to the unlimited expectations created by the mind.

Begin by practicing awareness of the aspects within your relationship that are influenced by these attachment based criteria. This will not be an easy task if your relationship is clouded with deeply-entrenched subconscious expectations.

Ask yourself some simple questions to reveal any attachment you're dealing with like:

Do I feel anger towards my partner because they are getting in the way of my career growth?
(Attachment to self - the island mentality)

Do I feel sad when my partner goes out with their friends?
(Co-dependent attachment - Feeling incomplete without constant attention/acknowledgement)

Do I get frustrated when they ask if I need help?
(Attachment to self - I'm independent; I don't need anyone)

Do I keep tabs on their every move; who are you texting??
(Co-dependent attachment - Lack of trust and the need to isolate the relationship from others)

Come up with some relevant questions that only you can answer. Unless you're in the rare minority, it's likely that attachment is more pervasive within your relationship than you realize. By bringing awareness to the attachments that are damaging your relationship, you can begin taking the necessary steps to counteract these relationship hurdles.

Identifying these hurdles is something that takes focus and active awareness. While you are in the throes of attachment, it is often difficult to realize you're guilty. In order to begin holding ourselves accountable and to discover the likely attachments hidden beneath the surface, change is necessary. In other words, do the opposite of what you have been doing within your relationship. If you spend every waking moment together, a weekend trip apart might expose your co-dependence. If you find that you feel bogged down by their constant nagging and your independence is being hampered, perhaps you have forgotten the many ways your relationship is encouraging your growth and actually *enabling* your independence.

Despite your independence (or lack thereof), we have an outstanding capacity to justify our narratives as *correct*. Most of the time we are wrong. Think about someone that proclaims complete and self-reliant independence. They still need others for many aspects of their existence. The opposite is true for someone that feels like they are lost without another. They are able to do many things independently but believe the lie that they are inadequate. By appropriately identifying your narrative, you will be able to experiment within your relationship and your personal life and discover where you have imbalance. What narrative have you created for your life?

Identifying these areas of weakness related to your attachments is only the beginning. The path to reaching a healthier balance in your relationship will be an ongoing process. Like many of my recommendations for achieving a healthier relationship, start with some small changes dependent upon the attachments you have identified.

For instance, if you need constant acknowledgement and reassurance that your partner still loves you, try creating some space in your texting correspondence. Do you really need to text them every hour of the day or could some space be a beneficial change?

If you take regular trips for work and avoid chatting with your partner for extended periods of time, would it really hinder your independence to take some time out of your busy day to have a short video chat?

I challenge you to be courageous and acknowledge the attachment that may be present in your life. This step can be one of the most difficult challenges in creating a healthier relationship, but if you are successful, the long-term benefits will become obvious.

Choose love, not the high

Whether you're in a new relationship or have been married for 50 years, challenges will continue to present themselves. Just like any skill in life, if you don't continuously improve upon your past methods, your skills will fade. This is equally true for a healthy relationship. If you are dedicated to growing and maintaining the relationship you desire, it is important to accurately and honestly evaluate your goals. Just like you would never build your house in the sand, it's important to get back to the roots of why you want or are in a relationship to begin with.

"Most people choose their careers with logic, and their love with passion. We have it backwards: choose your love with logic, and your career with passion."-Unknown

Understanding what you are looking for in a partner is paramount to your long term success. I'm not saying you should just leave your spouse if there are a few cracks in the foundation, but it is important to do an honest self-evaluation of your situation. I am a firm believer that almost anything can be repaired or built-up, but before that can happen, you need to do some deep digging and understand the source of your foundational problems.

It's important to understand the science of attraction. On a chemical level within the human brain, *falling in love* mimics a powerful high. We are literally on drugs. All of us. Unfortunately, love, and it's associated high will eventually come to an end. The butterflies will leave, the frustrations will begin, and your drug-seeking brain will naturally desire another love-fix. When you are in the passionate throes of a newfound relationship, you are blinded by the dopamine-like chemicals swirling throughout your bloodstream.

To combat this love-blinded-ness, I recommend that for any new relationship, you thoroughly vet the other person. It is important to have trusted friends and family members give you their honest feedback about your relationship. Carefully consider their perspective because, quite frankly, your brain is not to be trusted, and you're unfortunately high on love. But, a 'sober' friend or family member may help you to perceive your current reality a little more clearly. If there is a consistent theme of flashing warning lights and red flags coming your trusted advisors, you may need to re-evaluate and proceed with caution before moving forward in your relationship.

By recognizing that the pleasure-seeking reward center in our brains just wants to get high, we can rationally begin to gauge our relationships from a sober perspective. I want you to experience true love, not the superficial *feeling* of *love*. I don't think true love is a feeling. Rather, love is a series of focused and intentional actions that support a bond with someone you can tolerate. Yes, I know, *tolerance* sounds harsh. But, the harsh truth is that eventually even the happiest of couples get on each other's nerves and it's unavoidable. The things that you initially love about someone can quickly morph into annoyances without the proper perspective. I want you to be able to tolerate each other successfully and hope to show you how.

Love is choosing to treat the person you have agreed to share your life with the right way. Pillars of true love include: Respect, honesty, generosity, patience, and kindness. Notice, true love doesn't include: being served, fed, paid for, or clung-too. Let go of any ideas you have about love that can be traced back to attachment in any way. For instance, if you expect your husband to "be the provider", that is attachment to the idea of the man's responsibility to cater to you. I'm not saying it's a bad thing if your husband pays the mortgage, but it is when your love is conditional upon that expectation being met.

There is a fine line between a loving life together and an emotionally abusive contract. I repeat, let go of any outdated and expectant notions of love that you may have. You are solely responsible for your own joy and contentment in life. Let go of the idea that your partner is there to fulfill you. This dangerous illusion is propagated by the media and our self-serving society and leads to a false understanding of what defines a healthy relationship. If you believe that someone else will make you happy, you'll unfortunately be met with repeated let-downs. The minute that your relationship demands a service or ultimatum be fulfilled in your name, then your relationship has crossed from a love centric relationship into an abusive contract. If your relationship is all about you (or them), it's time for a change.

A fresh perspective on your current situation

I recommend starting with your own goals. For example, if you dream of becoming a world-renowned oceanic-photographer that has ambitious plans for traveling the world, a flexible relationship with a partner that also dreams of seeing the world is a great place to start. If you discuss your dreams with your partner but are consistently met with resistance and discouragement, that may be an indication that your foundation was never built properly. By beginning to identify some of your long term goals in life, you will have a better understanding of how your relationship meshes with your long term plans.

Gauge your current situation carefully. If you are currently single, but want to find love, have you considered self-improvement strategies before jumping into a relationship? If you feel trapped in a relationship that doesn't fulfill your needs, are you taking the necessary steps to improve it, or are you simply accepting the misery? If you know something needs to change, then you're in the right place. I'll be providing you with plenty of helpful self-repair ideas throughout this book for a quick tune-up. Try your best to remain humble and keep an open mind throughout this process because there is always room for growth. If you want to get the most out of your relationship, you owe it to yourself and your partner to make continuous growth a priority. Even successful and passionate lovers can benefit from adding new love skills to their repertoire.

Before going any further, I want you to reflect on some of your long-term goals and aspirations. Take a few minutes to write these down. Next to each of these ideas, I'd like you to identify **how** your current life situation supports these ambitions or goals. If your current situation **doesn't** support these ambitions, make sure to catalogue these points as well. By developing a clearly detailed list of your goals and which areas of your life are in alignment with those goals, you will begin to understand which areas of life are limiting or enabling your growth. Your long-term ambitions will be subconsciously swept under the rug by the busy-ness and repetition of your day-to-day routines unless you learn to become aware of why you are doing what you're doing.

Taking the time to become conscious of how your current life situation aligns with your long-term plans will help you to sort out where changes are needed. Effectively gauging your situation will have the added bonus of bringing renewed focus to the beneficial aspects of your life that may have been neglected. In other words, by weeding out the factors in your life that are slowing you down, your precious energy can be more effectively spent on your goal-supporting actions. This self-reflection is a great starting point for uncovering any obstacles in your life that might be secretly hindering your relationship progress.

In the past, I was guilty of desperately rushing into relationships. The hollow attempts to fill my empty heart led to greater heart-break down the line. I definitely needed a tune-up but needed to experience countless failures before I would realize this. I began to believe that relationships ending in tragedy was my eternal fate. Looking back on each of my failed experiences, I know that these failures were ultimately beneficial. While painful, each of my failed relationships taught me how to move forward with a clearer understanding of what it takes to create a lasting and healthy relationship. Even though consistent relationship failure was necessary for my growth, I know how badly failed relationships hurt and I'd like to help you avoid unnecessary heart-break. Instead, by approaching your love life with a clear understanding of your objectives and from a place of contentment within your own life, you will avoid many of the common relationship pitfalls.

If you are already in a relationship, but know that you need to do some self-repairs, it's never too late to make some tweaks. If your current relationship began with some poor choices or out of desperation, that doesn't mean your relationship doesn't have the potential to work out. Discovering your **reason** for wanting a healthy relationship will help you to sort out any of the difficulties you'll face along the way. With a solid reason, the motivation for making the changes you desire will naturally fall into place. Similar to the diamond: without the immense pressure that's necessary for development, if your reason for wanting love isn't strong enough, you're destined to fail. When you have a deep desire driving your actions to succeed in a relationship, working hard for that relationship will be seamless.

What do you want?

Before trying to find or fix a relationship, you need a firm grasp on what you're hoping to achieve. If you've made the common mistake of becoming involved in relationships before doing an honest self-evaluation, it's never too late to re-evaluate. It's important to understand *why* you're seeking a partner (or multiple) if you hope to have any success. Ask yourself some serious questions. When you open up an internal dialogue with yourself, you can begin to identify areas in your life that need an adjustment.

With a self Q&A session, you'll ensure that your destination is correctly entered into your love GPS. In the past, if I had taken the time to ask myself the tough questions, I would have saved myself a lot of time and hurt feelings. For instance, after a previous break-up, I quickly started dating another girl who was attractive but didn't check any of my other boxes. I hadn't even identified what my boxes looked like! If I had taken the time to ask myself, "What is important to me in a partner and am I ready to start dating?" I would have known from the beginning that it was a bad idea to become involved with that person.

Sometimes the answers are obvious. The most important first step of asking yourself the tough questions is often overlooked because of ignorant or selfish motives. I didn't know what I was looking for, and I definitely wasn't ready to start dating again. I didn't care. All I wanted was some instant gratification and temporary pain relief. Tough questions that I should have asked myself might have been:

- What kind of person would support my goals and dreams?
- Are there any personal hurdles that I'm trying to avoid or ignore by finding a partner?
- Am I capable of supporting someone else emotionally?
- What can I do to find more contentment in life before involving another?
- Do I really know which values are important to me in a partner?

Come up with your own self-evaluation questions. Hone in on any sensitive topics in your life and discover the root of your issues with honest questions. Don't rush this process. Understanding which areas of your life need change is a complicated topic and will continuously evolve throughout your life. Being able to accurately identify the source of your problems is an essential skill.

Another important question that will bring deeper issues to the surface: "How do you feel when you are alone?". If you are constantly feeling bored, lonely, and/or empty inside, chances are good that you need some self-healing before anyone becomes involved with your mess. It is important that you learn to enjoy your own company. If you live a lifestyle that is fulfilling; following your passions, constantly learning and growing, sharing meaningful experiences with friends and family- being alone won't be a problem.

This may sound narcissistic, but I love me. I enjoy my own company because I take action every day to *find* joy and push myself to become a stronger person. No one else is going to make my dreams come true, and no one else is going to spend more time with me than me. If you enjoy your own company then it's only natural that those in your life will also enjoy your company. But, keep that pride in check. Living your best life doesn't give you the green-light to be a stuck-up jerk. However, it does give you the green-light to share your passion and love for life with others.

Here are some ideas to help you can uncover important truths about yourself and your situation:

Q: "Do I have enough free time for a relationship?"
A: "Yes, but I need to re-organize my busy schedule and waste less time watching cat videos."

Q: "Am I looking for a long-term relationship?"
A: "No, I just want to have some fun. I think I will just stay single. I can still have a sex-life, but I will be honest about my intentions with any partners."

Q: "Do I want to have a family?"
A: "Yes, having children is a top-priority."

Q: "Do I want to have an open-relationship?"
A: "No, I want to find someone that is completely dedicated and loyal.

Q: "Do I spend too much money on drugs or alcohol?"
A: "Yes, I should stop drinking before I start dating again."

I repeat, take the time to figure out which questions you need to ask yourself. Write them down and add as much detail as you can. Don't cheat yourself by giving conservative answers. A thorough self-analysis will prevent a lot of potential problems down the line. You owe it to yourself to be a trusted advisor.

Imagine this scenario: You met someone while sloshed at the bar. You barely remember the first night you spent together. Fast forward two years; you're living together, you spend lots of money on gifts and romantic dinners. Everything is going perfectly; you really connect with this person, but you've just discovered a hard-truth. They never want to have kids. This is a complete deal-breaker for you. Both of your hearts will be broken unless you cave on your deep desire to have a family.

In this example you can see how powerful a thorough self-evaluation is. The massively heart-breaking scenario could have been avoided entirely. You never would have let the relationship go that far. When you create a frame-work of self-understanding through questioning your motives and desires, you set yourself up for future relationship success.

When doing a self-evaluation, ask for help. We have a tendency to deceive ourselves and a fresh perspective may lead to the answers you really need to hear. Trusted friends or family can provide insight into your current situation if you struggle with truthfully cataloging your set-backs. Share your self-questionnaire with someone you trust and brainstorm together on the aspects of your life that are getting in the way of the relationship you desire. Write down the revised edition that a friend/family member has helped you to create. It will become significantly less challenging to solve your problems once you have taken this important step. The healing and advancement of your relationship requires this.

You're not alone

Sometimes, the answers to your questions will be less obvious. Discovering the answers for your love life may require heart-break. The pain of sadness will expose intricacies in your character and sculpt an internal landscape revealing your true desires. That open relationship you thought was so perfect, left you feeling jealous and resentful. Learn from and use that pain to your advantage. Don't become a victim when you're sad because a relationship didn't work out the way you had hoped; harness that powerful emotion to create a relationship scenario that is ideal in the future. You've only failed in your love life when you let that failure define your future relationships. You're a success in your love life when you learn from previous relationship failure and apply that knowledge towards long-term growth.

Looking back, the relationship failures of my past ultimately became the most effective catalyst for the current relationship success I have today. During my most painful days, filled with hopelessness and anguish, I was unable to perceive the lessons that were being presented to me. Learning to accept our pain with an open mind and a willingness to learn from these moments is paramount to you achieving the relationship goals you hope to reach. In an interview with Will Smith when discussing his path to success, he wisely states, "Fail forward." Use every opportunity that presents itself as failure and learn from it. Without countless failures, you'll never gain the perspective you need to navigate the future with a clearer perspective. Keep this in mind the next time you feel hopeless or defeated. Your failures will become advancements if you let them be.

According to a study from Stanford University involving more than 4,000 participants, upwards of 70% of relationships fail within the first five years.

Break-ups become less likely with time

Annual risk of break-up, by year of relationship

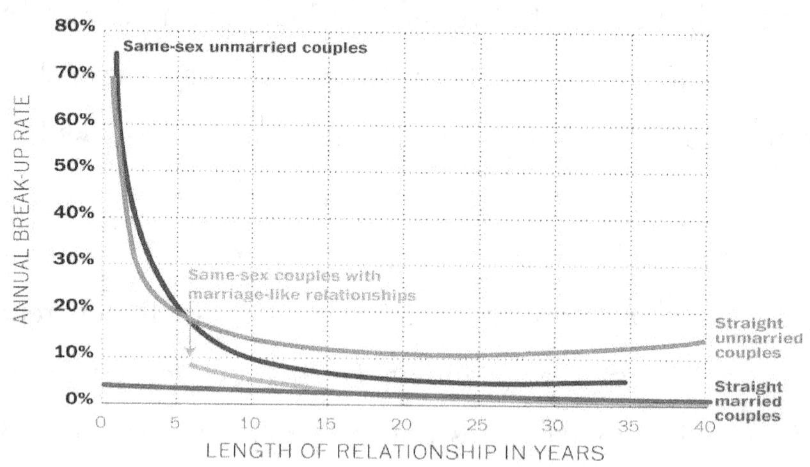

WAPO.ST/**WONKBLOG**

Source: Michael J. Rosenfeld, Stanford University

This staggering statistic is probably something you can relate to. Unless you're in the rare majority that married their high-school sweetheart and are living happily-ever-after, it's likely that you've had your fair share of love lost. In order to prevent repeated break-ups, it's important to decipher the reason behind such high-failure rates. While there are a million different factors that lead to disaster, I believe that these statistics would greatly diminish if every relationship started from a stronger foundation. In other words, if people spent the appropriate amount of time decoding their reason for wanting love, honestly evaluating themselves, and started taking the steps to create lasting self-joy first, then many of the couples surveyed would have avoided joining the 70% broken-heart club. In the following chapters, I'll outline a number of tactics you can implement to prevent just that.

If you aren't happy with your own life, how can you expect to bring happiness to another?

There are millions of people across the globe living in undeserved misery. We all want to have an enjoyable experience here on earth with our limited time, so it's of the utmost importance that we have the courage to take the necessary action to find that joy. Some people might blame their circumstances, their partners, or their empty bank accounts for their misery, but until we hold ourselves 100% accountable for our own happiness, we can never truly flourish in a relationship.

"Those who divorce aren't necessarily the most unhappy, just those neatly able to believe their misery is caused by one other person."

-Alain De Botton

Throughout my life, I have combated depression and other self-defeating mindsets. Overcoming and effectively managing these mental health hurdles is an important step in achieving relationship well-being. If you feel like your negative emotions are interfering with your ability to be the lover that you know you can be, it's important to take the necessary steps to heal yourself before you plan on moving forward in your relationship.

On my path to a more content perspective, I discovered several useful resources that ultimately led to a compassion-filled love life. If you are serious about improving your relationship (I'm guessing you are if you picked up this book!), then don't underestimate the importance of improving yourself throughout the process. Since adequately discussing self-improvement resources is beyond the scope of this book, I'll recommend a few that fundamentally changed my perspective. "A New Earth" by Eckhart Tolle, "The Subtle Art of Not Giving a F***" by Mark Manson, "A Liberated Mind" by Steven C. Hayes, and "Beyond Mindfulness" by Stephen Bodian.

Throughout my journey of self-discovery and personal growth, there were many times when I doubted myself. It was an internal battle driven by my crazy lizard-brain; preferring to wallow in misery rather than facing uncomfortable changes. I began removing toxic influences in my life gradually. This process of transformation took years, with growth still occurring to this day.

I was surrounded by unhealthy friendships that enabled my poor behaviors and was allured by the false-promises of various substances. I was completely miserable during this stretch of my early twenties, but refused to accept help because of pride and denial. Drinking and partying took priority over every aspect of a normal and healthy lifestyle. Time and time again, I would take a new job or find a new girlfriend only to eventually end up broken and alone because of my selfish behaviors.

Breaking this cycle of relentless self-destruction is difficult. Our egos will come up with a million different reasons to remain in that suffering. This primal thinking is based on the instinctual defense mechanisms programmed into our genetic make-up. Our minds resist any form of change out of a subconscious fear of the unknown. That's why it is so important that we take the steps necessary to become conscious of these underlying beliefs. If you can relate with this struggle in any way, then you have already taken the most important first step: the awareness of your crazy-lizard brain.

Once you have identified some of your limiting behaviors, you can begin to take **action** to resolve these issues.

If you can successfully overcome some of the barriers that are weighing you down, this transition will enhance your ability to become a more capable partner.

I also recommend seeking professional psychological help if you feel like overcoming some of your issues alone hasn't been working. Professional relationship counseling can be a valuable resource, but I recommend trying to implement some of the ideas presented in this book before you go that route. Therapy can be pricey, and you already have what it takes to create an ideal relationship, even if you don't know it yet.

It's never enough

I learned through naive expectations and some hard lessons that I'm the only one responsible for my happiness; No matter how much my partner does, it will never be enough to create lasting contentment. From date number one with the love of my life, I made it a point to find out if we could agree on the idea that our individual happiness was our personal responsibility first and foremost. This doesn't mean that I don't want to bring my partner happiness, but it is important to understand that I'm not responsible for their happiness. The excess of happiness that spills over from within is destined to be shared with your loved ones. If your internal cup is constantly drained, you're likely to be emptying your partners' cup in a vain attempt to replenish your own.

"Take responsibility for your own happiness; never put it in other people's hands." -Roy T. Bennett

On a fundamental level, it is impossible to be satisfied by anything outside of ourselves. Think about that gift you begged of your parents for months leading up to Christmas. You finally got that new bike you'd been wanting all year long. You did all of your chores, stopped picking your nose at the dinner table, and before long, you received that coveted gift.

Fast forward a year. Chances are good that the bike you'd wanted so badly has been collecting dust in the garage for months and you're already planning out a new wish list. This cycle of attempting to fulfill our happiness with outside temptations doesn't just apply towards the things we want. This habit of wanting the newest or shiniest next-best-thing is more relevant today with love than it has ever been. We have to strive with conscious effort to avoid the allure of temporary fulfillment and technological distractions if we are to discover just how much more valuable planning for the long-term can be for our relationship success.

Understanding and becoming aware of the attachments we have with our worldly-possessions reflects directly with our relationships. Instead of choosing to be happy with what we have, we have been sold the myth of materialism and conditioned to pursue pleasure indefinitely. This pursuit of pleasure and instant gratification can lead to a hollow existence filled with regret. Instead of seeing the beauty in the world and our relationships, we only look for what is missing.

If we allow ourselves to develop this perspective, we become blind to reality. Instead of learning to love each moment, we are lost in the rabbit-hole of attempting to fill the impossible-to-fill void that becomes our lives. Learning to shift out of the conditioned paradigm of our material world and the incessant drive for more stuff will take conscious effort. If you are ready to make this change and want to start seeing the world and love with a new set of eyes, read on.

Finding the silver lining in your life is not a small task by any means. At times, there won't always be one. Accepting that some days aren't filled with joy and excitement is part of the process of developing a more consistent peace and contentment. Learning how to weather stormy days and embrace your hardships with awareness will lead to a more balanced you. Rather than becoming a victim next time you're having a bad day, begin thinking with a solution oriented mindset instead. You may not be "happy", and that's fine, but you will spend significantly less time wallowing in misery once you make this change. Problem solving rather than dwelling will **always** get you through to the other side faster. Being able to hold your head up high during painful experiences is just as important as being able to recognize the beauty in your life. It requires diligent self-reflection and regularly reminding ourselves of our big picture love goals when we are tempted by anger or frustration. You may have an advantage if you already see the brighter side of life, but anyone can learn to develop this mentality. Through present awareness of your situations and a desire to change for the better, subtle day to day irritations and temptations will have a weakened hold on you and your relationship.

Take a step back from yourself

Cultivating the I'm-responsible-for-my-own-happiness mentality starts with taking a step back from your current life situation. Imagine that you are the contestant *and* one of the judges from American Idol. The singer (you) believes that their voice is a gift from above. The judge (also you, but somehow transformed into a scary version of Simon Cowell) says your singing is **terrible.** While trying to gauge our current life situations, we have to remember to be the judge, not the singer. Our "rational" and positive self-bias is misleading; it often distorts reality, leaving us deceived by ourselves.

"The Dunning–Kruger effect is a cognitive bias in which people with low ability at a task overestimate their ability. It is related to the cognitive bias of illusory superiority and comes from the inability of people to recognize their lack of ability." -Dunning & Kruger

I have fallen victim to this cognitive self-trickery many times in life. Disc-golfing, one of my favorite hobbies, is the perfect example. While watching the pro tournaments, I casually think to myself "I could do that, probably even better." The next weekend after finishing par for the day, I reflect on my previous self-deception. I missed many easy putts, and my drive was ~150 feet shorter than the pros. Reality played out very differently than the fantastical version my self-biased brain created. It turns out, reality is often very different from the lies we tell ourselves. That's why I encourage you to ask for help when cataloging your present state-of-affairs. If you know that things in your relationship seem a bit off but you can't pin-point exactly what the problem is, a trustworthy person in your life can provide the clear perspective.   When that person calls you out on your flaws, instead of being the defensive singer, compare and contrast opinions with a Simon Cowell perspective. You don't have to agree with their analysis, but have the courage to **try** and understand why they are reaching those conclusions about you.

If a friend or family member is willing to go through this process of discussing flaws with you, do your best to listen openly and resist the temptation to defend or make excuses for your past mistakes. Just listen and learn. The goal here is to identify your current issues- not to protect your ego. This step will help you to identify the **actual** self-flaws you were blind to because of your cognitive self-biases. Oftentimes, when faced with relationship problems, we waste a lot of effort fixing the wrong things because we never took this initial step to discover the source. It's not your fault, we all have the tendency to look at our lives through the distorted lens and want to think the best of ourselves. It's okay to think highly of yourself, but there is a fine line between self-confidence and self-delusion when it comes to the way you are living.

Once you begin to have a more thorough understanding of your flaws, I encourage you to take a look at other distractions that may be interfering with your love life. We are surrounded by the constant trappings of temporary pleasure. This is exponentially compounded by modern tech enabling instant gratification through hook-up dating apps and other shallow social media platforms[1]. The culture of instant gratification has undermined countless relationships because it encourages a subconscious belief that we always need more; this subconscious belief creeps in and infects our relationships. Instead of learning how to compromise and practice forgiveness, we throw out the old relationship at the first sign of trouble. This is a result of the instant gratification programming; knowing that a new lover is only a tinder swipe away. We need to break out of these patterns of

---

[1] Modern tech can also help you stay connected and/or find love; I'll discuss some of modern tech's advantages later on.

relationship-destroying selfishness if we ever hope to find a love worth holding onto.

I'll never forget one of my favorite hospital patients while working as a Nurse Aide. Bill was a kind-hearted gentleman that had a sharp mind unencumbered by his frail body. We often discussed philosophy and other topics relating to human nature. As our friendship grew, I felt comfortable enough to share some of my relationship woes with him. He was successfully married to his high-school sweetheart for more than 60 years and had obviously mastered the craft of love. I was desperate to learn how it was possible. When I asked him the secret to such a long-lasting and seemingly joyful relationship, I was anticipating a complicated and mind-numbing explanation of the inner-workings of love. To my surprise, he replied "Simply treat every-day like it's your first day together. If something breaks, you fix it. You don't throw it away."

This simple approach completely transformed the way I started behaving in relationships. I was guilty of having flighty tendencies; I had become a victim of the instant-gratification mentality. I wanted the perfect relationship without any of the work. The painful components that are required to fix a relationship were brushed aside because it was easier to quit. Don't be a victim to that quitter mentality. If you find someone that is highly compatible with you and cares as deeply for you as you do for them, it is worth the effort to mend that relationship when things will inevitably break. After mending issues within a relationship, a depth of understanding between the two of you grows. From the struggles that you overcome, you will learn that you can count on each other no matter what life throws your way. Instead of jumping head-first into ideas for fixing your relationship, let's start by identifying if you are a victim to instant-gratification programming like I was.

Let's start with a small practice. Identify one area of temporary gratification in your life right now that either steals time or resources away from you. Instead of buying that new pair of socks that just popped up on your Instagram feed, start a mini-savings account designed for romantic endeavors. When you consciously shift your time and resources towards things that benefit your partner, rather than your temporary pleasures, you will begin to cultivate an attitude of genuine compassion towards your loved one. When being generous with your time and energy begins to become second nature to you, temporary desires will become less appealing. Learning to be less selfish leads to intentional compassion that will have a profound and long-term impact on all relationships in your life.

How often do you start something and give up before you've completed that goal? I'm guilty at times. Let's see if I can finish this book. I struggle with the temptation to move on to the latest and greatest new idea. I want to blame the culture I was raised in, but I know that I am the only one responsible for learning the patience and resilience required for accomplishing anything worthwhile in life. While I occasionally falter and revert back to my old selfish patterns of instant-gratification, through self-awareness and practice, I have become much more willing to push through difficulties in life. I want the same for you.

You might find yourself inspired by something and decide that you're going to accomplish a goal. Well, what happens after the path to that goal becomes harder to travel down than you'd anticipated. Do you say to yourself that this is too hard and start trying something else instead? Your goal was abandoned because you felt that it just wasn't worth the pain and effort. This is a by-product of instant-gratification tendencies and it's important that you become aware of how you behave whenever you are faced with a challenge. If you are able to keep your nose to the grind-stone during challenges situations, any challenges you face in your relationship will be handled from a stronger position. Learning to persevere and continue pushing towards your goals and dreams will take conscious effort.

Bill made it seem so easy when he said just fix it when it breaks. Well, back in Bill's day, they didn't have Amazon Prime and had to solve their own problems. The fact that we live in such a throw-away culture makes it all the more challenging for us. It is imperative that we learn to shed the temporary pleasure mindset and begin taking effort to think like Bill. How would you fix your relationship if throwing it away wasn't an option?

Understanding love languages

Before taking action towards a stronger love life, it is important to identify you and your partner's love languages. Even if you are currently single, these key concepts will help you connect with friends and family on a deeper level. After years of experience with marriage counseling, Gary D. Chapman wrote "The 5 Love Languages."[2] Essentially, our love receptors are all unique. We all respond to love differently, and if we aim to become effective lovers, we must be fluent in our lover's language. Gary identifies the 5 love languages as follows:

- Words of affirmation
- Quality time
- Receiving gifts
- Acts of service
- Physical touch

In my relationship, I utilize each of these different expressions of love. Through trial and error, I have found that physical touch, words of affirmation, and quality time were the most meaningful expressions in my relationship. Take a

---

[2] See References.

few minutes to think about how each of these languages speak to you. Do you feel like your partner is regularly wasting money on gifts, when you'd rather just spend some time cuddling on the couch? Do you feel like your partner has resentment growing over the multiplying dirty dishes? Subtle changes in the way you show appreciation and practice daily love in your relationship can have a profound influence for positive change.

I don't recommend the trial and error approach to discovering each other's love languages. I spent a lot of money on gifts, thinking that would impress her, only to later realize that the sentiment wasn't as powerful as I had intended. Instead, I prefer a much less questionable route; simply ask your partner what really makes them feel appreciated and loved.

Another less obvious path to discovering your partner's love language is through listening. Oftentimes, you can easily decipher what is important to their heart through their complaints. The next time your partner is upset, they may be providing you with a helpful hint. Are they regularly complaining about the dirty dishes you leave behind? Then, show them your love through the *act of service* by doing the dishes. Do they complain that you work too much? They are quietly informing you of their longing for more *quality time*. Figuring out which love language speaks to your partner is essential.

The same goes for which love language speaks to you. Instead of assuming that your partner should know how to please you, be direct. Tell them what kinds of affection warms your heart. When you take the guesswork out of your relationship, you'll hear less complaints and share more genuine love.

Trust is a priority

I was recently watching the show "90-Day Fiancé" and identified a major recurring point of tension: lack of trust. The couples featured in this show have found love with people from other countries. Most of these relationships developed quickly while on a vacation or through online sources. In order to avoid a challenging distance relationship and the complex citizenship requirements of the U.S., the couples opt for a K-1 (fiance) visa instead. These temporary visas thrust the couples into a 3-month marriage deadline. If the couples don't wed before the 3-month visa expiration, they will be forced to separate and return to their country of origin.

This rushed timeline creates a hurdle because many of these relationships haven't had the adequate time necessary for the development of trust. The show perfectly illustrates how essential the trust component of any relationship is because this stressful timed experience bypasses many of the necessities required for a healthy foundation. Time and time again, disagreements spring up over basic relationship fundamentals that were glossed over. Initially, each of these couples begin with high hopes and good intentions, but inevitably, the reality of their poor foundation becomes evident as the constant conflicts become pronounced.

The misguided hope and good intentions leave them blinded to the fact that any strong relationship requires the appropriate amount of work upfront. While there are exceptions and a *love at first sight* scenario can lead to a life of happiness, these instances are high-risk and unlikely to succeed. If you have the option to establish a healthy framework built upon trust before becoming overly involved, take that route instead. The complicated components and inner-workings of love life will be realistically manageable when a steadfast degree of trust is established prior to commitment.

Unconditional love that can withstand the daily hardships of life is built upon trust. The early phases of a relationship often make it glaringly obvious if the trust factor hasn't been established appropriately. Some early warning signs revealing a lack of trust in your relationship might include: unwarranted jealousy, questions about your whereabouts, monitoring your social media/texts, or lack of communication/openness.

When you have established a secure level of trust with your partner, you won't have a need to be jealous, worry about what they are doing, or feel the need to watch their every move. Reaching this point in your relationship should be a priority. When you feel secure in your commitment, you'll be able to face future relationship troubles with confidence knowing that your partner will always have your back. Developing this level of security with your loved one takes time and should be given the attention it deserves.

Through consistent honesty and openness in all aspects of your relationship, trust will grow naturally. Trust doesn't develop overnight, and if you've ever given your partner a reason to doubt your integrity, this process can become prolonged. Instead, create a trusting relationship from the beginning by taking every opportunity available to practice integrity.

To build stronger trust within your relationship start with a welcoming attitude and open communication. When your partner feels that they can openly share their feelings and wishes with you, they won't have a need to keep secrets or become resentful. If your partner is feeling emotionally neglected or desires more physical affection, instead of cheating or lying, they will freely communicate their needs to you. Listen without judgement and before long, your partner will trust in you for all things. This attitude of openness will lead to closeness, a feeling of security, and an eagerness to share their life with you. You must be a source for your partner to confide in. If they can come to rely on you during the hard times without feeling judged, trust will become definite and unbreakable.

A mutual trust is the bed-rock to all other areas of growth and will prevent unnecessary anxiety. Your partner won't have to worry that you're lying or keeping secrets because you've proven yourself through your open and honest attitude. This behavior will motivate your partner to reciprocate that honesty and in turn, trust mutually grows. The key to maintaining this is consistency with your actions. No matter how uncomfortable complete honesty and transparency can be, setting the integrity standard high should become your priority. Express this to your partner and clearly explain why you value honesty so highly.

This idea is equally relevant if you are already in a trusting relationship. Each and every action you take that involves your partner can either solidify or undermine the current level of trust. I challenge you to take note of each and every deceitful action or thought that crosses your mind. If you have developed a snake-tongue and lies slip through your lips regularly out of habit, do your best to bring awareness to this side of yourself. Begin writing down any lies you catch before they leave your mouth. Carefully analyze the lie and try to decipher the root cause of that deception. Did you lie about taking the dog out because you didn't want your partner to think you were lazy? Did you lie about sending that important work email because you were neglecting your job but wanted to impress your boss? Whatever the lie is, become aware of it.

Oftentimes, we think the things we are hiding are egregious and unforgivable sins, but in reality, being honest in these moments would often make our lives less stressful. This can be a complicated hurdle if you have used deception to your advantage throughout life. Exceptionally adept liars often get by for a while, but no matter how sneaky they are, eventually the lies creep to the surface.

What may seem like a harmless white lie or minor broken promise can lead to relationship destruction if you allow deception to gain traction. If there are currently any secrets or lies haunting your relationship, reveal these things to your partner. Your crazy-lizard brain will tell you to keep lying out of self-preservation. Don't listen. If you create a habit of hiding behind little lies, it won't be long until reality brings out the truth and feelings are hurt beyond repair. One lie can lead to another, and before long, the lies will grow in magnitude and create separation in your relationship.

Ultimately, a lie only exists because of the false pre-tense that it is useful. Perhaps, you think that the truth would embarrass you or that your partner couldn't handle it. While being honest can be painful during the reveal, this temporary upset is a price worth paying for the overall benefit to your relationship. By openly sharing all of the hard-to-talk-about issues with your partner, you will prove to them that honesty is your top priority. Being a person of integrity and honor takes courage.

The importance of establishing a strong foundation of trust cannot be stressed enough because building up trust takes time; breaking down trust can happen rapidly. Reduce your chances of breaking the trust you've worked so hard for by holding yourself accountable **each and every** time you are tempted to lie, cheat, or deceive your partner. The temporary self-protection is not worth the potential damage these selfish behaviors reap.

Trust Exercise: Think about an uncomfortable secret or a strange/embarrassing habit that you have. Ideally, this secret or habit is something within the light-hearted realm, such as a nose-picking habit. Once you've come up with your idea, I want you to share this with your partner. The idea here is to open the door for discussion and to let your partner know that you value them enough to share everything with them. By creating this exclusivity and by sharing your secrets with your loved one, they will likely return the favor. Getting to know the nitty-gritty details about each other should be fun, and if you can laugh about the embarrassing aspects of life, then sharing the more serious things with each other won't be so cringe-worthy. Establishing a comfortability and rapport with each other will lead to lasting openness.

Later I'll discuss ideas for cultivating appreciation for your partner and help you to come up with some realistic expectations that will make the entire process of trusting each other seamless. When each partner's needs are consistently met, trusting each other will become second-nature. Becoming the rock-solid partner that you know you can be will take focus, courage, and a commitment to a higher standard of living.

Love and money

A major point of tension for many relationships is finances. Since the aim of this book is to help you remove tension from your love-life, it's important that we discuss the money side of love. You might think this contradicts the previous mention of "we can't be fulfilled by anything outside of ourselves", but unfortunately, money indirectly influences every aspect of our well-being and our relationships. While true peace and contentment come from a deeper place, an acknowledgement and understanding of the financial realm is necessary if we hope to maintain a lasting relationship.

On my journey to find the silver lining in life, much of my growth came from studying and understanding the connection between wealth and overall contentment in life. I have come to understand: it's true that money won't bring you happiness, but money will provide you with the tools required to live to your ultimate potential. When you are taking courageous action to pursue your biggest aspirations, it's only natural that you have a deeper satisfaction in life. Through accumulation of wealth, you are enabled to live more fully through the *freedom of your time*. When you are able to choose how you would like to spend your day rather than being forced to punch a clock, you unlock opportunities in life that bring out the best in you. Ask yourself this: If you had 10 million dollars deposited into your bank account today, what would change? If you would live differently than you are right now, then it's quite possible that your true potential is being limited by financial forces.

For a long time, I had a poor relationship with money. I thought that trying to get "rich" was a selfish endeavor. I believed the myth that "money is the root of all evil". This myth is simply a lie developed and perpetuated by our society and by leadership in order to keep the masses impoverished. If a population remains in poverty, the people are more easily controlled. I won't get too deep into the psychology of poverty, but there are forces at the top trying to keep you poor because they understand that wealth is a powerful tool for freedom of time.

You deserve to be rich. Not only does a healthy bank account provide peace of mind, but it also encourages your growth. With a healthy balance sheet, you are able to pursue passions that would otherwise be neglected. If you never had to worry about money again, imagine how much more time and attention you could spend on the ones you love and the hobbies you enjoy. Fights that start over worries about the bills being paid would transition into enjoying each other's company instead. Wouldn't you rather worry and fight less, while enjoying more time with your loved ones?

If this concept seems like a disconnect from the relationship world, I challenge you to analyze your current financial affairs and think back to a time to when money has interfered with your love life. I can think of more than one instance where financial woes interfered with my love life. For example, I would often work overtime at a job I despised just to make ends meet. This led to sacrificing valuable time and energy that could have been spent with the person I loved.

As well as absorbing the majority of my precious waking hours, I was drained from a long day's work. I would finish a 12 hour shift at the hospital only to come home and crash on the couch like a zombie. I was not an effective partner. I was constantly tired and had very little energy to spend on my relationship. Instead of bringing my best-self to the table every day, I was drifting along in quiet desperation, wishfully thinking that eventually it would get better. My relationships suffered because I remained in a state of hopelessness based on the belief that I would always be poor. I was a victim to the rat-race-for- life mentality with no end in sight.

I encourage you to read the book "Rich Dad, Poor Dad" by Robert Kiyosaki. In this book, he discusses tactics for removing yourself from the job/self-employed world and transitioning into the business/investing world. If you really want to live to your fullest potential and be the best partner you can be, you must learn how to get your ideas and money working for you, rather than spending your precious time coasting in a meaningless job that will never earn you enough money to realize your dreams. You deserve to be rich.

Think about something you're really good at. Instead of thinking about the process of becoming rich as a complicated business equation, simply think of it as a way your current skills might be able to help others. Ultimately, the best businesses in the world exist because they effectively make their customers' lives simpler. Can you think of a way to add value to others or simplify a process that needs to be improved upon? When you begin to think like a value adding creator rather than a victim of circumstance, you'll find that hope and joy for life is an automatic by-product while changing your life in the process.

In the classic self-help book "The Science of Getting Rich" by Wallace D. Wattles, he outlines the importance of the creative/value adding mindset. When you apply yourself in any business or love endeavor, only apply yourself from a helpful and giving mindset. By remaining in the creative/value adding headspace, you are operating at a higher frequency that will draw others with similar mindsets to you. This may seem like a stretch, but there is a power that comes with contributing to the world around you with the grateful and value-adding mindset. You will no longer feel like you are competing with the world; you are working symbiotically with the world. When you begin to believe that the world is full of abundance rather than feeling like you never have enough, opportunities will begin to materialize in your life.

I have personally tested this theory out and I know that the power he speaks of is true. The more value I add to others, the more willing they are to share their value with me. A cycle of abundance emerges that self-replenishes and manifests into opportunities that are conducive to fulfilling your true potential. When your focus becomes solution oriented, you waste less energy dwelling on the hurdles in your life. We are all connected in this universe, and when you optimize your opportunities through this shift of mindset, your life will continuously improve and your distant dreams will become reachable.

There are many other ideas presented in the materials mentioned above that will help you cultivate mindsets for growth. The value of developing a grateful, optimistic, and abundant attitude cannot be stressed enough when trying to change your finances and life for the better. By creating a purpose driven life by challenging yourself to become your best self, you are positioning yourself to be an amazing lover. By creating value in others' life through your efforts, you will find renewed passion in your life that is contagious. Others will want to be near you. Others will care about you because you have learned to care so much for them. As your mentality solidifies into a more grateful state, love will pour out of you and heal those around you. I'll go into detail later on ways that you can practice gratitude more successfully.

There are many money making opportunities available to you right now that require little experience or know-how. If you agree that finances have created problems in your past or current relationship, then figure out a way to increase your cash-flow. There is no excuse for letting your bank account get in the way of becoming your best-self and being the best partner you can be.

I currently work a full-time job assisting Anesthesiologists in the operating room. While this strain on my precious time is significant, I acknowledge that by taking the steps necessary to grow my wealth, I will eventually be able to live life entirely on my terms. I enjoy my work, but I would rather be able to take vacations or pursue other hobbies as I see fit. Instead of listening to detrimental thoughts like: *I can't, I'm too busy, this is too hard,* I have discovered some extracurricular money making opportunities so that I can eventually be more free, which will enable me to become a more available and compassionate partner.

Take action today. Figure out at least one opportunity that will begin relieving some of your financial stress. When you start living with a mindset focused on creating abundance for others, you will find abundance for yourself in the process. How much time do you spend watching T.V., procrastinating, or drinking with friends? Any activities that are slowing you down could easily be replaced with a side-hustle.

It doesn't have to be complicated. Just figure out what you are good at. How can you share that knowledge with others? When the primary goal is to help others grow in life, the money that comes along with that giving of yourself is just the icing on the cake.

For example, writing this book is one of the avenues I've chosen. I have transferred wasted energy (watching television in the mornings on the weekends) into writing this book. After brainstorming ideas for how I could add value to others, I ended up here. I struggled with this change. Every fiber of my being resisted this transition away from "comfort". But, the desire to live up to a fuller potential in life trumped the desire to be temporarily comfortable. The same will apply to you. If you truly want to change your life for the better, you have to be willing to make the sacrifices necessary.

Here are some examples of opportunities that you can start today:

- Online/Retail arbitrage (search for deals then resell on Amazon, Ebay, Craigslist - I use TacticalArbitrage.com to find great deals) Look up Bill Stenzel on

YouTube.com, he has some courses on arbitrage that are very thorough, but not free.

- Freelance Work (there are platforms available for everything from writing gigs to graphic design work - I use Elancer.com and Upwork.com)

- Learn how to trade stocks (I use Webull and TDAmeritrade's platform: ThinkorSwim). Check out the books "How to Day Trade/Swing Trade for a Living" by Andrew Aziz and "Secrets for Profiting in Bull and Bear Markets" by Stan Weinstein.

- Create an online store to sell anything (I use Etsy.com, but other platforms like Shopify.com enable you to create an online-storefront easily) A fulfillment service like Printful.com allows you to upload your designs onto their platform and they do the rest. You link your online store to their site, and they will print your design onto t-shirts, mugs, and other accessories and ship it to your customer. You can focus on your designs while they handle all of the materials and logistics.

- Create a YouTube.com channel or start a podcast. Share your knowledge and make $$$ through advertising, affiliate marketing, or by selling a product/course. There are countless free tutorials on YouTube.com on how to make a YouTube channel profitable while you simultaneously share your knowledge with the world! Win-win.

- Start any business. There are countless ways to fund your business idea with no cost to you. GoFundMe, Kickstarter, and IndieGoGo are a few popular crowdfunding platforms. What problem can you solve and how can you do it better than someone else?

Money challenge: Sit down with your partner and create a financial plan for your relationship. While this might be an uncomfortable subject to discuss with your partner, it is necessary to iron-out any financial details and expectations early on in the relationship. I recommend creating a thorough list of your collective monthly incomes, expenses and variations. Even though I don't recommend creating a budget (They don't work in my opinion - it's better to automate your savings/investments), I do recommend you have a thorough understanding of where each and every dollar you spend is going. Once you have a thorough and detailed list of your incoming/outgoing numbers, collectively decide if anything on this list conflicts with your long-term financial goals.

Outlining a financial plan is designed to reduce conflict in the long run. If you are a big saver, but your partner is a big spender, going through this process can bring light to any potential problems brewing beneath the surface. By uncovering any areas of weakness in your shared financial situation, you can decide together on the best path to get back on track. Do your best to keep emotions out of the equation and focus on the facts. Clearly define your mutual goals, and create an automatic savings plan to reach those goals. This understanding will significantly reduce conflict down the line.

Once you have established these financial guidelines, debates over unnecessary purchases will gain less traction since there is a pre-agreed upon plan. For example, if you both decide that 300$ a month spent on entertainment and eating out is okay, fights over those extra-curriculars won't be an issue. If you decide that one person is entirely responsible for all financial decisions, that is fine too. Just make your expectations clear at the beginning and do your best to keep your emotions out of any financial discussions.

No matter your financial well-being, finances should never be an excuse for tension in a relationship. In my relationship, we split the major costs of living such as housing, groceries, and utilities, but beyond that, our money is ours to spend as we wish. We established those guidelines when first moving in together, and have yet to have a single fight about finances. We hold ourselves accountable for all personal bills and understand that our individual financial situations are our responsibility but know that we can come to each other if an emergency or surprise expense comes along.

Your situation may not be as simple, especially if kids or an unexpected job loss mandates a financial pivot. Remain flexible and willing to compromise. There may be times in which all of your best laid plans fall to pieces. You might lose a leg or your house or the clothes off of your back. Establish new guidelines and find a solution without **ever** letting your temporary situation interfere with the health of your relationship. Struggles, overdue bills, and a mountain of stressors will lure you into lashing out, but never let anger over a situation turn into anger towards your partner. When financial worry inevitably happens, figure out a way to transfer that stressful energy into productive money-making energy instead.

It's all about the personality

What kind of personality and attitude do you portray? Would you want to spend time with you?

I used to be a jerk. I was angry, sad, and cold hearted. I was always blaming the other person when my relationships inevitably ended in disaster. I was a serial dater, jumping from relationship to relationship thinking that maybe I was just consistently unlucky. It turns out I was very wrong. *I* was the problem. My expectations were outrageous, my standards for "beauty" were delusional, and it was all about me. I was a disfunctioning alcoholic that was too blind to see how blessed I was. Family, friends, and co-workers all tolerated my company because they could see the potential I had, even when I couldn't. This didn't last. I lost many of my friends and was fired from multiple jobs because of the self-loathing and drinking. Fortunately, my family was supportive and unconditionally loved me throughout these dark years. I believe their continued support was one of the catalysts that helped me to overcome this destructive period in my life.

Long story short, I would not have wanted to date me. Looking back on that period in my life, I realize that the majority of my relationship woes could have been easily avoided. The solution? Become someone that I would want to be around. I began to study the habits and lifestyles of people that were enjoying their lives. Time and time again, I found that the people who discovered contentment and passion in life also cultivated personalities of kindness, generosity, gratefulness, patience and other attributes that I admire. Instead of continuing to dwell in misery, I began taking steps to develop these character traits.

If you can relate with the darkness I've experienced, then you're in good company. If you've struggled with depression or other debilitating emotional issues, it might seem like there's no light at the end of the tunnel. I promise you that no matter what you're dealing with, it is possible to change your perspective if you have the desire to overcome your situation. Being able to view life with an optimistic outlook is vital to your relationship success. Nobody wants to be with someone that is constantly draining energy and moping around.

Through exercise, surrounding myself with uplifting friends, and by focusing on *how* to become a more joyful person, I was starting to become the person that I wanted to be around. Once I successfully made these necessary changes, the quality of my relationships improved accordingly. When you exude an uplifting energy, people will be drawn to you. People living joyfully will take notice. Kindness loves company. Once you successfully shift your perspective towards the blessings you have in life, your friends will be many, your relationships will be lasting, and you will have renewed hope for each day.

What steps are you currently taking to become the person that you would want to spend time with? On my journey of continued growth and the pursuit of lasting joy, I've discovered some important action steps:

- Exercising daily (preferably outside)
- Learning something new (I am currently reading a book each month for the rest of this year)
- Practicing gratitude daily (using "thank you" and "I appreciate you" regularly in conversation when appropriate)
- Cultivating friendships with energizing and creative people
- Maintaining a clean home (peace of mind and an act of service to self)
- Scheduling focused time for my relationship daily

- Meditating centered on breathing exercises and other sensory inputs
- Increasing my earning potential (By-product of adding value to others)

Decide for yourself what you can do each day to grow towards your long term goals while simultaneously warding off self-defeating emotions and attitudes. The hardest part of adding growth opportunities into your daily routine is decoding which areas are holding you back. If your relationships have continuously failed time and time again, working on yourself first is the likely remedy. Throughout this book, I'll provide several strategies to help you upgrade your personality and ultimately have the fulfilling relationship and life that you deserve.

Discovering your passions

Within all of us, there are some unchanging truths. We all want love, acceptance, and to feel like we are making a meaningful impact in the world. Finding out what passions call to your heart can be a life-long search. Recently, I listened to a motivational speech by Joe Rogan[3] in which he refers to the perpetual state of unhappiness as, "quiet desperation." In this speech, he discusses the vast amounts of untapped potential in humanity that is being stifled by the demands of daily life. Instead of taking the time to discover what is truly important in life, we often opt for the normal/comfortable/boring route because of perceived safety through familiarity. This deceptive comfort ultimately leads to sadness and unfulfilled potential.

It's imperative that we diligently seek out new experiences and discover new passions so that we can find contentment in life. If you are excited for life each and every day, any relationship you have will share in this joy. By freeing yourself from the cocoon of dreadful malaise, you will begin to see life with an optimistic outlook.

---

[3]Joe Rogan Motivational Speech: https://youtu.be/SZEo1KFjTn4

You can take action today to begin discovering your passions. Opportunities to expand your horizons are readily available and simple to discover. Although, trying new things can be an intimidating prospect if you are deeply entrenched in your comfort-zone. Your comfort-zone is **not** where you want to be. Start small. You will find that growing into new passions is an easy way to enhance you and your partner's life.

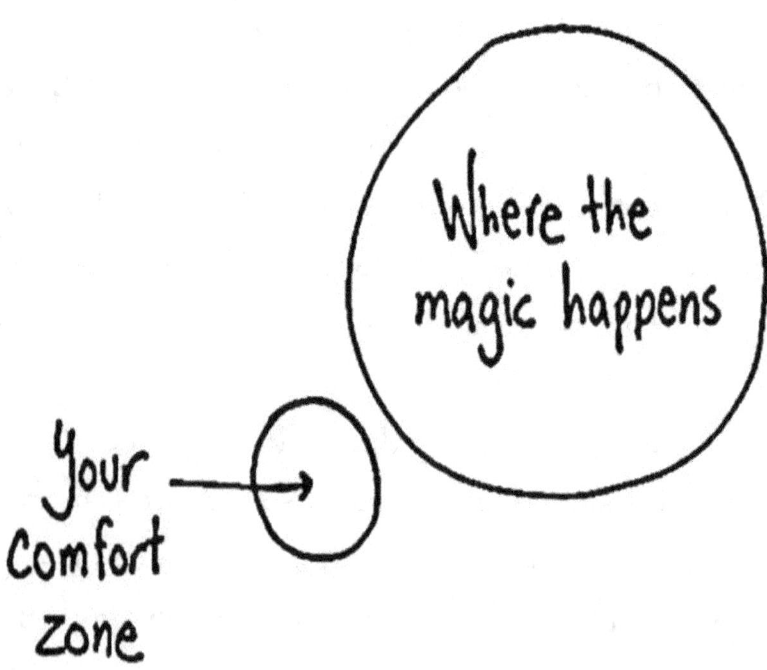

I recommend searching through your local paper to find some events or classes that are outside of your comfort zone. If a fearful thought arises, do your best to ignore that defeating thought, and focus on the goal here: discovering a new passion that will expand your horizons and enrich your relationship.

You often don't need to look very far for new opportunities. Strike up some conversations at work; try asking your co-workers what they like to do for fun. Perhaps your boss likes to go on kayak trips, and happens to have a double-kayak for you and your spouse to borrow. Reach out to your friends and ask if they have any suggestions for fun date ideas. Do some online searches for exciting opportunities in your area. The options are limitless if you have an open-mind and are ready to experience a richer love life.

Perhaps you already have some exciting passions. Let's begin digging deeper into your interests by writing down some of these ideas. Alongside each of your passions, carefully consider why each of these ideas enhances your life. Be completely honest with yourself and add as much detail as you can. The more vivid and complete your descriptions are, the more useful these ideas will be later on when deciding which passions are a priority for you.

Some examples of passions that are a priority for me would include:

- Exploring nearby trails and parks. I love the outdoors and feeling the connection with nature. At least a couple times each month, I will explore an area that I have never been. I really like to do this without a specific route planned, and I discover so much about the world around me without having to travel very far.

- Tasting new foods and learning how to cook unique dishes. I feel that through food we are taken on trips across the globe. The sensations of different spices and combinations provide a unique experience that increases my appreciation of food.

- Challenging myself to continuously grow and try new things. I have decided to pursue a path of growth through good books, selective friendships, and an active lifestyle. I have been writing down my goals, and taking action every day to continue on this path of healthy change.

Once you've identified some of your passions, we're going to do an exercise of the imagination. Going through each of the passions you've listed, imagine what your future or current partner's involvement with that might look like. For example, if one of my listed passions, such as running, is a high-priority for me, having a partner that encourages that passion is essential. If my partner were a couch-potato that lacked any sort of motivation, this could conflict with my active lifestyle in the future. While there are obvious exceptions to this concept, it is necessary that once you have prioritized what is important to you, you remain steadfast in your passions despite the consequences. After all, life is short, and if you're surrounding yourself with negative energy that is preventing you from reaching your full potential, then it is time to reflect on what you are willing to compromise.

As well as supporting you in your passions, it is vital that you equally share in supporting your partner's goals. If your booming art career demands 60+ hours of your week, but you expect them to show up at each of your new gallery showings, then make sure you are also willing to make similar sacrifices for them. There is no such thing as *too busy* for the ones we love. If this seems to be the case for you, I encourage you to look over your passions list again and decide which priorities in your life may need some re-adjusting. If you look over your typical weekly schedule, more likely than not, there are gaps throughout your busy week that are filled with time that could easily be spent on your relationship instead.

Now that you've identified some passions, take action

It's time to put those ideas you've come up with into action. The most joyful times in my life have often been related to overcoming a challenge or learning a new skill that I believed to be beyond my abilities. If you really hope to have a healthier and stronger relationship, it is necessary for you to cultivate an environment of growth that will ultimately lead to a fulfilling love life.

"You will find joy in overcoming obstacles." -Helen Keller

Pick one of your passions. Any passion. Let's say, you're excited to learn more about sustainable living and would like to start a garden. Normally, you might just do a search for some gardening tips online and buy a few potted plants for your deck. Instead, harness this idea to grow deeper in your relationship by turning this passion into an amazing date idea or continually shared activity. In most cities, there are local botany clubs or guided nature tours through botanical gardens that will give you some great ideas for getting started. Learning to nurture life together can have a significant impact on your relationship. Whichever passion you select to implement into your relationship, the focus should be on growing together while accomplishing something new.

Get your lazy lover off of that couch, and take them with you to that hands-on nature tour and learn how to plant some flowers. You might be surprised at your results. By taking some initiative, you can build something together that will bring you shared pride while simultaneously uncovering new joys in life. Gardening might not be the best option if you're dealing with average-joe brown-thumb, but having the courage to take a dance lesson or private cooking class could ignite some new sparks in your relationship. By taking this focused action you will learn more about your partner, illustrate how much of a priority they are in your life, and break out of draining routines that are disastrous for relationships.

No big deal if they don't like all of your ideas

Don't expect every passion you bring to the table to be a shared passion. Your partner may seriously disdain walking through an uppity art gallery, but it's important to attempt some new ventures together. If your partner is reluctant to go on some new adventures, start by showing interest in activities related to some of their passions before trying anything too extreme. When they see that you are open to their passions, they will be more receptive to your suggestions in return. By challenging each other to experience new things, you will discover new aspects of your partner while simultaneously developing a deeper appreciation for each other.

Simple changes in your day to day routine can give you similar results. If you are paired in an exceptionally routine relationship, you'll have to be creative with your add-ons. Resistance to change is a natural response, so don't expect your partner to go along for the ride automatically. The last thing you want to do is develop unnecessary tension in the relationship when changing things up because it's only natural for your partner to initially resist change. Instead, start with subtle changes that can be worked into the routine. As your partner becomes more comfortable with the smaller changes, in time, bigger changes that you hope to implement will be met with less resistance.

Some simple examples from my relationship include: writing out a list of ideas for new recipes that we plan on cooking together, visiting new disc golf courses, and going for walks with the dog. While these subtle changes may seem overly simple or quite plain, these little changes are quite effective when hoping to grow closer with your partner. We learned better communication through shared cooking, we encouraged each other with the new golfing challenges, and we had uninterrupted quality time on our walks. By making little changes to your routines, this will lead to greater willingness and openness to future changes. Adding excitement into your love life doesn't need to be complicated. Start today and figure out a few ways to mix up the monotony of daily life.

Fish Bowl Passion Challenge:

Cut up some scraps of paper and write down interesting ideas for dates, quality time, or adventures. Be creative. These should be simple ideas that you can do at home or without having to leave your hometown. Ask your partner to come up with some ideas too. Without looking at each other's scraps, throw them into a bowl and mix em' up.

Pick a day each week where you both have some free time and select a random scrap from the bowl. No matter what the scrap says, you both have to agree to go along with the idea! This is a wonderful relationship exercise for learning about each other's passions while adding some excitement and creativity into your love life.

Using habit to empower your relationship

If you find that getting your partner motivated to mix up the routine is a larger obstacle than you had imagined, consider changing up some relationship habits. Learn how to master the art of encouraging positive change through unlearning old habits. I'll teach you how, and if that seems like too much work, you can always just bribe your partner to go on that adventure with you! If this seems extreme to you, consider the alternative: a boring life together.

In the book, "The Power of Habit" by Charles Duhigg[4] He discusses some of the inner-workings related to habit. Everything we do in life is consciously, or subconsciously, done for a reward. Think about the tasks in your life that you absolutely dread doing. All of these things in life are tolerated because we anticipate that the end goal is worth the effort.

Whenever we hope to sneak a new habit into our routine, there is a simple method to accomplish this goal. Charles Duhigg illustrates habits using a looping cycle consisting of: Cue -> Routine -> Reward. In order to use habits to our advantage, we first must understand which habits we'd like to

---

[4] See Bibliography

replace. If you are a smoker, and your spouse hates the smell of tobacco, replacing this habit would significantly improve relationship health, as well as your own. I was smoking half a pack of cigarettes daily prior to applying the technique described below. Rewiring your habits isn't as complicated as you might think.

Identify a habit in your life that is interfering with your relationship. Examples might include: Watching too much T.V., an online-shopping addiction, overindulgence in alcohol, or a tendency to become angry when confronted. Each of these examples have a specific **cue->routine->reward**. Let's break down the T.V. example since I'm sure many of you can relate with this one:

The cue: Dinner is ready and you are hungry. **The routine**: You watch the news while you eat, and then watch another two hours of your favorite sitcom. **The reward**: You feel full and relaxed.

To effectively change this habit, instead of trying to replace the entire cycle, simply insert a new routine. We can trick our brains into compliance by keeping **the cue** and **the reward** the same. This method is extremely effective because it prevents our crazy-lizard-brains from defensively resisting the change. We effectively trick our brains because all we're really after is the reward. After inserting the new routine, the new habit-loop would look something like this:

The cue: Dinner is ready and you are hungry. **The (new) routine**: You eat dinner while sharing quality time at the dining room table with your spouse. **The reward:** You feel full and relaxed.

Now that you understand how simple it is to modify the habits in your life, refer back to the list of habits you created earlier. Start with the most detrimental habit and break it down into the three phases; **the Cue, the Routine, the Reward.** Again, like the other principles in this book, start with a small and easily achievable change. Changing the patterns of our lives will take time. Keep your eyes on the reward and your chances for rewiring unwanted routines out of your life will come with time.

Identifying the cues for certain habits can be difficult. Many of the cues that trigger the habit cycle are subtle, and often operate within your subconscious awareness. You may not even realize that you're in the midst of a habitual routine, until it's too late, and you've already missed the cue. When I made the choice to stop smoking cigarettes, there were many triggering cues that I needed to become aware of. Boredom, stress, time of day, and social activities were all cues. At the root of each of these cues there was a state of discomfort, albeit, presenting itself in different ways. What I ultimately discovered after an honest internal evaluation. My reward for smoking was alleviation of temporary discomfort.

Once I had identified my cues, I decided on a replacement routine. In this case, I decided meditative deep-breathing exercises and exercise could easily fit the bill and provide the desired reward of alleviating discomfort. I didn't succeed immediately, but as I continued to become more aware of the triggers, the process of using meditative-breathing and going for a run instead of having a smoke became the new routine. Be patient and forgive yourself if you struggle with these changes because rewiring your brain takes significant perseverance and a strong desire to change.

Focus on the reward if the routine is dull

There will be times when you are faced with frustrating aspects in your relationship. If you look at these frustrating obstacles with an eye on the prize, your anger will diminish. Focusing on the reward (the reason) you are doing something will help you to develop patience and a long-term outlook. Once you understand this concept, the difficulties in your relationship will be viewed with a more forgiving perspective and less selfishness.

To shift your focus towards the reward, and less on the dreaded routine, here is a simple challenge. Write down every tedious obligation in your life. Include anything that is a source of frustration in your life. Your list might include: Chores, family gatherings, business meetings, or responding to emails. Once you've come up with some irritating obligations in your life, make a separate column labeled *end results*. If doing the dishes is on your list, the end result would be a tidy kitchen and a clean work space for the dinner prep. If tolerating business meetings made the list, then the end result might be job security and a healthy bank account.

By analyzing why we do the things we do in life, we can begin to have a more joyful attitude when trudging through the tedium. In my experience, this transformation happened while I was washing the dishes. I felt regular frustration when I would wake up to a sink full of dishes. A bitterness and resentment emerged as I thought, "She just doesn't respect that I prefer a clean kitchen and is always leaving a mess!" I didn't want to let such simple tasks create tension in my life, so I decided to change my perspective. Instead of perceiving this *mess* as a source of frustration, I began to consider this as an opportunity for me to show kindness in my relationship.

When I do the dishes now, I am focused on the end-result of a clean kitchen (for me), and a show of kindness towards my partner (for her). This change of perspective from dwelling on the dreaded task to the satisfactory end result reduced my overall frustration, while simultaneously providing a compassionate and useful expenditure of energy. It's amazing how such a subtle shift in awareness can create an overall win-win situation for everyone involved.

Many times, the reward we seek is subtle and may go unnoticed. When deciphering which habits are preventing contentment and creating tension, it takes an aware mind to uncover the truth. Realizing which rewards you're seeking out can help you to break down each individual frustration into manageable segments. Get to the root of your frustrations and you will see that almost every situation can be transformed into a pleasant experience with the knowledge that your rewarding end-result awaits you.

Make the time, don't wish for it

Finding the time for each other can be a challenge in any relationship. If your work-life balance is way out of proportion, this may seem like an impossible task. But if you are willing to do a little creative maneuvering, it is easier than you think.

I recently read a book called, "The 4 Hour Work Week" by Timothy Ferris. I learned all about managing my time more effectively for greater efficiency in all arenas of life. One of my favorite sections relates to how our typical eight-hour work days are generally filled with a majority of fluff and a minority of real productive work. The same can be said of how we spend our free time. If we aren't careful, sitting down for a 30 minute Netflix session can quickly morph into an entire season binge.

By recognizing when we are losing precious time to these passing distractions, we will become more aware of how we could be spending that time more productively. Once you've discovered which areas of your free time could easily be transferred to growing your relationship, you'll find that finding time for each other was never as difficult as you may have previously believed.

Similar to creating a financial budget, I recommend you create a log of how your time is spent throughout the day. Do this for a week minimum, since your availability and schedule will fluctuate day-to-day. This may seem like a tedious process, but it's important that you learn to become accountable for your wasted time. There is often dead-space between activities in our schedules that can easily be transformed into productive usefulness. For example, instead of listening to the news for 15 minutes before work every morning, you could spend that time writing a heart-felt love note. The 15 minutes that were wasted watching the news has now been transformed into a meaningful expression that will brighten your partner's day.

Do you feel like you are constantly busy and find yourself wishing for more free time? Practice becoming aware of these little distractions in life. Constant phone alerts, idle time in between scheduled events, and incessant email follow-ups can steal the precious moments of your life. These little moments add up; it's time that you can spend more effectively towards your relationship growth.

Our will-power is weaker than we believe. By utilizing simple tools to rewire our conditioning and develop new habits to maximize our time, we can begin to overcome our time wasting patterns. By learning self-discipline when it comes to setting relationship goals, blocking out time in our days for our loved ones becomes a habitual process. Instead of reading through spam emails, a regularly planned heart-felt message to your loved one inspires a pleasant foundation for the rest of their day.

Again, I want to emphasize the necessity of keeping this change simple. If you are overly ambitious with your new goals from the beginning, your inherent tendency to drift back into old patterns may surface. Start with a few simple tweaks to your schedule that will enable more productive use of the wasted gaps in your day. For example, a lunchtime notification on your phone reminding you to send a heart emoji. Simple, yet effective.

I recommend accomplishing the most *tedious* goal for your day first. By accomplishing the most arduous task first, anything else on your goal list will become less intimidating. By completing dreaded tasks earlier in the day, it frees up your mind to focus on the things that are truly important.

This simple life hack changes the way you perceive your schedule and propels you into effective momentum that lasts throughout the day.

For example: I decided to get up earlier on the weekends to let the dog out and brew the coffee. This small change required minimal input, yet produced powerful results. I used to dread getting up early, and cherished sleeping-in on the weekends. I would lay in bed apathetically with no clear purpose defined. By establishing a few minor tweaks to the start of my day, the precedent is set for a continuation of that effective momentum. The action of getting up earlier to handle mundane tasks is now a conscious habit that keeps me on track for the rest of the day. This habit mutually benefits my relationship since my partner is able to sleep-in on the weekends, and I am consistently more productive.

Once you've come up with a log for how you've been spending your time, find some gaps and pencil your partner in. Even if nothing else in your schedule changes except transitioning fluff time into productive time spent on your partner, their sense of feeling valued will increase exponentially. Scheduling a block of time each day for your loved one should be a priority if it wasn't already. It could be ten minutes, or it could be two hours. It doesn't matter. The point here is to be intentional and consistent with setting aside time **every day** to focus on your relationship. Turn your phone off. Turn the T.V. off. Focus on what you know is important: **your time and your relationship**.

Opportunities to give in your relationship will become more obvious once you've taken the step to schedule your partner in. Besides spending more time with your partner, think of some ways that you can make the most of those moments. While brain-storming, try to envision what struggles your partner may have. By envisioning what difficulties your partner is dealing with on a regular basis, you will automatically become a more generous and empathetic partner. Take intentional action today that will alleviate some of the pressure from your partner's shoulders. By reducing stress in your partner's life, you both benefit tremendously.

If you never take the trash out, do that. If a family birthday is coming up, go out and buy the card. If you leave your muddy shoes in the hallway, stop. By accomplishing something that tailors to their wants and needs, your partner will feel deeply cared for and acknowledged. Implementing these little changes into your daily routine will lay the foundation for growth in other areas. If you apply the *finding the time* advice from the previous chapter, taking action for your partner will be much less of a chore since you've discovered all of that free-time.

"I have found that among its other benefits, giving liberates the soul of the giver." -Maya Angelou

When you give, do so without expectation. The entitlement mentality is a devious menace that can sneak up on initially heart-felt generosity. What starts out as an act of kindness can quickly morph into darker emotions if left unchecked. Similar to *focusing on the reward*, the rewards of generosity come in many forms. When thoughtless giving occurs, selfish desires fade away and lose their luster. The rewards may present themselves in the form of contentment, peace, or through direct appreciation from the recipient. Receive these rewards of your generosity without allowing pride or self-righteousness to creep in. This sounds simple in theory, but to truly become a compassionate giver, you will have to remind yourself regularly of the *reason* you are giving. By keeping the focus centered on the aspects of your relationship that you're grateful for, staying on the path of selfless compassion is the natural result.

Sometimes you will give and no one will notice. If you're in a relationship that's very one-sided, constantly giving of yourself without any recognition will eventually wear you down. Feeling underappreciated at times is normal but can become a problem when these feelings aren't acknowledged or addressed with your partner. Guard yourself from allowing anger or resentment to grow by having the courage to discuss any feelings of "being taken for granted" with your partner. Continue to give of yourself without expectation, but take note if lack of acknowledgement becomes a consistent theme after you've tried to address the issue.

It's important to distinguish the difference between your generosity and when you're being taken advantage of. If you find that you're being taken advantage of in your relationship despite your best efforts to resolve the problem, this could be a major warning sign of a one-sided relationship. If you feel like you can relate to this situation, the sooner you discover the reason for this behavior, the better.

A common theme in relationships that leads to resentment is the silent giver. Throughout the course of a relationship, it's very likely that initial generosity is appreciated and recognized. Unfortunately, one of our double-edged traits as humans is our ability to adapt to circumstances and establish new baseline norms. This adapting process gradually turns into accepting recurring kindnesses (such as the dishes being done every night) as the standard. Eventually, the chore that you started doing out of love for your partner becomes **expected.** Instead of feeling underappreciated and letting this emotion fester, address your partner directly if you'd like them to help around the house more.

It might seem like a chore to constantly talk about these things with your partner, but it's necessary to regularly recalibrate your relationship and establish a healthy baseline. It's okay to ask them for help with the chores they've started to expect. Let them know how it makes you feel and why. If you're worried about being perceived as a nag, start off the conversation by asking about their needs first.

For example, "Is there anything I can do to take some stress off of your shoulders? I know you've been busy at work lately, but I feel like I'm the only one cleaning up after dinner and some nights I'm tired from work too. Would you be willing to help clean a couple nights each week? In return, I'll get back to rubbing your shoulders before bed like I used to." By acknowledging your partners' wants and needs before bringing up requests, their guard will be lowered and chances of reception improved. After you've had the discussion, don't forget to be thankful for their willingness to help and adjust to your needs.

The generosity must be a shared responsibility. Perhaps you've been taking your partner for granted in subtle ways without realizing it. Just as you must hold your partner accountable with shared responsibility, you must remain equally open to compromise as well. If your partner is always taking out the trash, show them you appreciate their efforts by taking on the burden from time to time. By remaining conscious of the little things that are easily taken for granted and by lending a hand in all arenas of life, you're one step closer to keeping mutual appreciation at the forefront of your relationship.

Do you have unreasonable expectations?

It's best to keep expectations to a minimum. Even though it's a priority that you find someone who shares in your dreams and supports you unconditionally, let's reflect back to an earlier point: we are the only ones responsible for our own happiness. If you are satisfied with yourself, you will find that accommodating the desires your partner has will be less of a chore. There won't be a void in your heart that you are hoping to fill from the outside. Rather, you will have so much excess to share from within that going above and beyond will become second nature to you.

This doesn't mean that you should have **no** expectations for your loved one, but begin to identify which of your expectations are selfish desires versus which expectations are truly important to the health of your relationship. For instance, if you both work long hours, but you are the only one preparing dinner and doing the dishes, it's a realistic expectation that they are willing to help you a few nights out of the week. However, if you expect a massage every night after work, it might be an unrealistic expectation based on selfishness. By figuring out which expectations are fair for both of you, it's much easier to prevent any resentment that may be quietly bubbling up beneath the surface.

Write down some of the expectations for your relationship. My list would look something like this:

- I expect my partner to remain loyal.
- I expect my partner to treat me with respect.
- I expect my partner to be open and honest with me when they feel wronged or frustrated.
- I expect my partner to encourage me when I feel strongly about something.

Notice that none of the expectations listed here are unrealistic. All of these ideas are centered around simple ideas that are easily accommodated and mutually beneficial. By having healthy expectations that you communicate clearly with your partner, you'll have a solid understanding of areas in your relationship that need some work. If your partner has a pattern of bottling up whenever you try and discuss what's on your heart, encourage them to open up with you by honestly expressing why this is important and necessary to you. By becoming vulnerable and admitting that clear communication is important to you, chances are good that they'll begin to open up. Never blame someone for not meeting your outlandish expectations if they never knew what those expectations were to begin with.

As humans, one of our weaknesses is developing the victim mentality. When someone wrongs our ego, we often create a narrative of being assaulted. Following this false narrative, the pain that you consequently project outwards is expressed through passive-aggressive undertones or an overtly abusive reaction. Instead of openly communicating why we feel that we've been wronged, our ego's natural response is to assume that they should have known better and to immediately react with retaliation.

Your partner cannot read your mind! Days and days of resentment over doing the chores begrudgingly builds until the inevitable avalanche of suppressed passive-aggressive rage comes raining down upon your unsuspecting victim. Your clueless husband may have foolishly thought that you liked to fold his clothes. He is constantly enraptured by the shiny football flashing across the screen, oblivious to you regularly passing by with a full laundry basket, again failing to offer a quick, "Thank you." While it is possible that your partner is just cold and unkind to your labors of love, it is more likely that they are unaware of the issue at hand.

Explain your expectations to each other! Many recurring issues torment otherwise happy couples because they never take the time to detail how they prefer to have things done. When realistic expectations are paired with open and honest communication, this solution acts as an investment towards the prevention of future resentment and tension. When you build a foundation of clearly explaining expectations to each other, World War III, the home edition, can be prevented before the first shot is fired.

Come up with realistic expectations

Once you've figured out some of your realistic expectations, it's equally important to figure out which expectations need to be slashed from the record. I'd recommend sitting down with your partner and taking turns writing down some of the things you do for each other, and discover if these things are being taken for granted. Be thorough and create a detailed outline of every aspect of your daily lives. By carefully considering all of the seemingly mundane things, some of the little day-to-day tasks that have been taken for granted might make the list of unrealistic expectations.

By exposing the expectations in your relationship that are creating unwanted tension, you can begin to open up a dialogue about what needs to change. This will assist in creating alignment of expectations that are mutually agreed upon. Don't force this process, since a perception of *nagging* can occur. These expectations will constantly evolve as you grow in your relationship. Through clear communication, any new relevant issues that emerge will be handled appropriately. With a new understanding of each other, I can guarantee that chores that were once taken for granted will start getting the appreciation they deserve.

*Be aware of the little things, because they are the
big things*

A major factor leading to divorce and breakups is a lack of appreciation. So many fights could be prevented if there was more appreciation shared. I have first-hand experience in the healing powers of the three little words, "I appreciate you!" When your partner's hard work and efforts are noticed, their feelings of self-worth and value sky-rocket. Even if you are completely satisfied with your own existence, we still have a genetic need to feel appreciated. On a cellular level, we cry out for that simple acknowledgement, and it's one of the easiest things we can implement into our relationships right now.

The act of appreciation towards our loved ones starts with awareness. By actively noticing all of the little things you are grateful for in your relationship, all the little quirks that used to irk you will seem like non-issues because your relationship mindset begins to shift. Just like a bright light blocks out the darkness of a room, maintaining a constant attitude of appreciation towards your partner will block out those previously resentful or angry thoughts.

Start small. Just like any bad habit, it can take a while to undo the thought patterns you've developed throughout the course of your relationship. I'd recommend starting a journal that you keep by your bed-side. Every night, write down one thing about them that you are grateful for. Even if you just had a fight over the dog puking on the couch, I don't care, focus on what you are grateful for. The key here is to maintain consistency. This practice is designed to help you cultivate a habit of being aware of why you are in the relationship to begin with. This can be hard when you are in a toxic relationship, but that is an even better reason to put some serious effort into developing this habit. [5]

After one week of doing your daily gratefulness exercise, share this with them and ask that they do a week or two of nightly entries as well. After you've both come up with some great ideas, talk about them with each other. Let your partner know that this is really important to you, and be thorough in your discussion of these topics. Provide examples in detail for each of your entries so that your partner understands the

---

[5] See Chapter #15 for further discussion on appropriately dealing with toxic relationships.

depth of your feelings. By developing this expectation of being grateful towards one another, you'll begin to see your relationship shift along with your new-found mindsets.

It's easy to lose sight of the original reasons we fell in love. Perhaps you've become numb to your relationship or are so deeply entrenched in your own worries that your partner is just an after-thought at this point. Focusing on thoughts of gratitude towards your partner is a path out of this numbness. Practicing gratitude is an exercise in awareness and will begin to shift the perspective you have for your partner.

In the past, I was a victim of my relentless negative thought patterns. When something upset me, I'd go deep into the rabbit hole of self-destructive thought patterns that were multiplying faster than I could push them away. These self-centered thought patterns prevented me from being a caring partner. I had forgotten why I had fallen in love. When thinking back on this period in my life, I now realize that I was living in an unconscious dream state; a prisoner of my thoughts rather than practicing awareness for all of the blessings surrounding me.

By bringing awareness to the thoughts that stifle your relationship when they initially spring up, we can center ourselves in the moment and escape that vicious cycle. The next time you notice you're lost in another downward spiral of negative thinking, take a moment to center yourself through deep breathing or by focusing on a sensation in your body that is happening right **now**. The simple act of bringing your attention to the moment and simply reflecting on gratitudes will instantly break you free of the mental prison. Learning to become aware in the moment will not only bring you peace and happiness, but it will reflect powerfully in your relationship.

Let's consider two likely relationship scenarios.

Scenario #1: Lost in your vicious thought patterns:

You woke up on the wrong side of the bed today, and the coffee you spilled on your new jacket was just another blow to your horrible start to the morning. Anguish and dread swirl throughout your mind as you cruise robotically towards your prison cell. You pull into the work parking lot and notice your parking spot has been stolen by your not-so-favorite co-worker, Nancy. Isn't it enough that you have to hear her prattling on all day while you're trying to focus on your reports? You hear from more than one of your bosses about the typos in last week's reports, but just smile and pretend like everything is fine. You've been staring at the clock all day and just wish you could coerce the minute hand to move a little bit faster. The clock slows with each passing second as you dream of the weekend and its temporary freedom from this torment called work.

Nancy can be heard drumming on about a new shade of pink nail polish as the incessant sound of her nail file grates against your brain. It's only Monday and you think to yourself, *"I can't take this any longer."* It's finally five o'clock and you drive home in a zombie-like trance swarmed with self-defeating thoughts of self-pity and dread for the upcoming week ahead. I wish it was Friday.

Back in the house, you begin reliving your awful day. When your spouse walks in the door, you're lost among your miserable thoughts and fail to recognize her arrival. While staring off into nothing, you think, "What a bad day, I just can't catch a break. What an annoying boss, they're too blind to see just how much I'm contributing. Nancy's such a nuisance, she doesn't even realize how awful she can be, I wish she would just shut up for once."

You finally lift your head and realize that your wife is there. She looks concerned. Instead of a warm greeting and your charming smile, you immediately spew the contents of your wreck of a day all over the place. After thrashing her with this gut-wrenching negativity, you grab a beer and slink off into the living room. You soak mindlessly into your armchair for a few hours in a desperate attempt to find solace in the mindless images flashing across the screen.

Scenario #2: Practiced gratefulness and awareness throughout your day:

You wake up on the wrong side of the bed today, but lie silently and focus on your breath for a few moments. You can hear your spouse breathing quietly and remember how lucky you are to have such a beautiful woman in your life. On your way to work, you reflect on the journal entries you shared with each other last night. You feel a sense of relief knowing just how much she appreciates you. The car ride is smooth today and traffic seems to be flowing with every turn of the wheel. You continue your focused breathing exercises while simultaneously smiling at the beautiful spring blossoms emerging along the side of the highway. You feel calm, motivated, and are looking forward to your productive day ahead.

As you pull into the parking lot, you notice that Nancy has taken your parking spot again. You remind yourself about your goal of getting back into shape this year, and smirk at her car as you stroll from the back of the parking lot. You're 300 steps closer to meeting your daily steps goal and notice how fresh the air tastes this morning.

In the office, your boss casually mentions you missed a few things in the report last week. Instead of feeling attacked, you take a look at the report and realize that he was right and thank him for showing you what needed to be fixed. Your boss smiles at you and says, "That's the kind of attitude we like to see around here. Most of the time I just get dirty looks when I bring any mistakes up around here. I appreciate your professional attitude and strong work ethic."

Back at your desk, you can hear Nancy talking about her new nail polish and remember that your wife just got some new pink shoes and might like a shade like that to pair with her outfit. You step over to Nancy's cubicle and ask her, "What brand was that Nancy? Sorry to eaves-drop, but I think my wife would really appreciate something like that. You always seem to be keeping up with the latest trends."

She tells you which store she went to, and suddenly gasps, "Oh, I wanted to apologize to you! I hurt my foot doing yard work and wanted to park a little closer. I should have asked you first, but I remembered you sounded all excited last week when you were talking about your new work-out routine. I figured I could help you out by making your walk in a little longer!" She laughs and points at my gut that was trying to bust out of my tucked in shirt.

You return a charming smile and scoff, "Thanks to your forced parking lot exercise regiment, my gut isn't long for this world! And thanks for the tip. I really think she'll appreciate that I'm starting to show some interest in her style for once. I've never taken the time to notice the little things before, but I'm really starting to see just how powerful a little intentional giving can be."

"Yeah, most guys just don't get that." Nancy sighs, "If only every gal was as lucky as yours is, I think there would be a lot fewer broken hearts out there. Anytime you need some love-pointers, let me know. I've been through a lot of bad relationships and so many problems could be avoided if people started thinking like you do."

Back at your desk, you reflect on how wrong your first impression of Nancy was. You've made a new friend and found an insider for future relationship advice. You ease back into your comfortable office chair and take a moment to bring your focus back to your breath. You feel clear, calm, and focused. With a delicious cup of coffee by your side, you turn on your computer and start working.

After fixing the reports, and adding some other information that you'd overlooked, you look up and realize it's already 5 o'clock. This was one of your most effective days yet. On the way home, you reflect on the productive day at work and make a quick stop at the general store to grab that nail polish. You remain calm despite the horrible traffic and use this extra time to continue practicing your meditative breathing techniques.

When you get home, you notice some dirty dishes in the sink and take care of them. As you're putting away the last plate, you hear your wife coming in the door. She looks stunning in her new pink outfit, with a smile to match. You look into her eyes and give her a deep hug as you remind yourself just how lucky you are. After she tells you about her busy day at work, you pull out the nail polish that perfectly matches her outfit. She beams. You know she feels appreciated and loved. Instead of shrinking into the couch like you used to do, you share a bottle of wine together and enjoy the evening with a heartfelt conversation and renewed passion that you haven't felt in years. You're loving your life and every moment that you're blessed with.

Shifting your perspective

In the above scenarios the days played out very similarly but minor tweaks to perspective made all of the difference. By looking at situations throughout your day with gratitude and opportunity rather than judgement and frustration, the things that used to get under your skin lose their power.

In the classic self-help book, "The Science of Getting Rich" by Wallace D. Wattles[6], gratitude is a central component for any type of success. Another key component of this resource is that through visualization of the life you desire, the universe will begin to bring these desires into material reality. Whether you believe in mystical interference from the universe or not, a key take-away is the overarching principle of maintaining gratefulness and shifting your focus towards a view of continual abundance. Awareness of just how fortunate you are in any given moment will raise your frequency.

Wattles compares these different frequency states as the competitive state (What can **they** do for me) to the creative state (What can **I** do for them). When you are operating in the

---

[6] See Bibliography

creative state, which is maintained through gratitude, your purpose is centered in finding solutions that are constructive. When you know in your heart that there is a wealth of abundance constantly available to you, and so many things to be thankful for, excitement for life takes center stage.

When you apply the principle of gratefulness in your relationship, improvements will seem to appear magically. The farts in your relationship may not start to smell better, but you begin to handle challenges with a renewed resilience. I equate this process to lifting the grey veil from your minds-eye. The world seems a little brighter, and hope flourishes in ways that you have only dreamed of.

I know this concept may seem a little outlandish, but I challenge you to put this idea to the test. I don't subscribe to any ideology or methodology unless I have experienced the results for myself. I have been putting this practice into action for the last four years, and I can honestly say that I have never felt such a persistent contentment in life.

The gratitude we share with each other has a compounding effect. Just like every action has an equal and opposite reaction, practicing diligent gratefulness towards your partner will be appropriately returned in-kind. Instead of a cycle of resentment or frustration developing, which leads to more and more resentment or frustration, a cycle of giving for each other develops. As you continue to feed into this gratefulness spiral, the positive momentum prevents toxicity of the past from resurfacing.

Your obstacles only appear to be massive

No matter how trivial or difficult the task at hand is, a strong desire to overcome often leads to success. When I was in college, studying for the Physical Therapy Board Exam, I felt a nagging sense of failure before I had finished reviewing the first chapter. I refused to listen to those thoughts. Instead, I began to cultivate an attitude of perseverance knowing that if I diligently studied and put my mind to the task, I would prevail. Three short months later, I passed the exam on my first attempt despite the nagging thoughts of failure that were constantly looming.

Think about an obstacle you've encountered in life or in your relationship. When you are in the midst of an obstacle, doubt has an uncanny ability to creep in. It's as if all of your fears are roaring at you; every noise is drowned out by the thundering defeat echoing throughout your skull. This is why I challenged you to take a step back from your current situation earlier on. It's important that you are able to view your difficulties with a big-picture perspective. If you continue to view your problems from the same flawed vantage point that you started at, you're destined to continue suffering.

In "The Subtle Art of Not Giving a F*ck" by Mark Manson, he presents a valid theory for reframing your life. If we listened to all of the detrimental whisperings of our minds, the outcome would be perceived failure. This belief that we are *losing at life* in any form is self-created myth. By reframing your life from perceived failure into the acknowledgement that you are already winning, your obstacles begin to lose their power over you. You may not be living up to your ridiculous and outlandish standards for fame, fortune, or success, but you're succeeding whether you realize it or not.

When you put in the effort and want something bad enough, you will always reach the end goal. It may not be the exact outcome you had imagined, but the end result is an advancement of self. Think about everything you've achieved so far. The job you hate so much is the realization of a goal you once had. When you went in for that interview, you won. By reframing our current issues from the perception of failure into acknowledgment of accomplishment, we begin to see the world more clearly.

Take responsibility for your perspective and current situation. Any stresses you're currently tolerating are *all* stressors you're willing to tolerate. Our willingness to rationalize or blame outside forces for our dilemmas is a shallow attempt at deflecting the responsibility for the choices we've made. If you say your job is intolerable, stop tolerating it and find a new job! It's a grievous disservice to yourself if you continue to push off this responsibility. Stop lying to yourself and admit that your problems are only still hanging around because you have tolerated them too well. Take the action required to make your situation tolerable. Any second you spend dwelling on a problem is wasted time. Figure out which avenues you can take to reach your desired end goal: a more content existence.

The little things challenge

Similar to the journal entries focused on cultivating gratitude that you started earlier, the next exercise in relationship growth will be a personal challenge. The little things challenge will have big results for your relationship.

To begin, simply pick an object near you. It can be a coffee mug, a pen, or your phone. Once you've picked out your object, I want you to imagine everything from its creation up to the influence it has upon your life. That simple pen may have a seemingly minimal influence on your life, but you can't deny that the pen has value. It enables you to write a friendly note to your neighbor, provides something to nibble on when you're nervous, or helps you finish your kid's homework.

While imagining the entire creation process of your object from start to finish, consider all of the different resources and businesses that were involved in that process. While imagining its many different capabilities, consider other powerful aspects of that object you may not have considered. The simple pen in an adept artist's hands can create beauty out of thin air.

This stretch of the imagination may seem like a pointless endeavor, but it is a necessary step in mastering the art of appreciating the little things.

Take some time to go through this imagination process with other nearby items. The goal of this exercise is to train your mind to view things from a new perspective. Using every-day objects makes this exercise even more effective. When you learn to find value in the most common of items, the things in your life that are truly important to you will take on a new depth.

After you've practiced with some items, I want you to go through this imagination process while focusing on thoughts of your partner. Think about how many lives they've influenced. Think about the first time you met and how stunning they looked. Think about all of the gifts they've given you. Think about some of the best memories you have with them. Just like you imagined the creation of the pen, I want you to imagine how much joy and value they've added to your life. That time your car broke down and they came to pick you up. The day you were yelled at by your boss and they patiently listened. The way they comforted you when you were having a bad day.

When you are going through this process, try to create strong visualizations of these memories. Feel the emotions attached to those moments and make them come alive. Reliving these experiences through imagination is a powerful mental exercise that strengthens your ability to appreciate the little things in your relationship. The next time your partner goes above and beyond by cleaning the house, you will be primed for gratefulness automatically.

Now, reflect on something that they're directly or indirectly doing to influence your life for the better. They might be sitting on the couch drinking a beer right now. You may not feel like they are adding value to your life, but perhaps your perspective just needs a little tweak. For instance, before they were in your life, you desperately longed for the companionship you now have. You wanted someone that was laid-back, down to earth, and enjoyed watching movies. All of your criteria have been met, and yet you have a thought of resentment towards them because of perceived laziness. By remembering to appreciate the little things in your relationship, your heart will be shielded from the negative thoughts towards your partner.

It will not always be easy to find the silver lining in your relationship. That's why I call it the little things **challenge**. If it weren't a challenge, it wouldn't help you grow. Let's discuss a few different ways you can start implementing this idea into your relationship.

I recommend setting a notification on your phone to remind you a few times throughout the day to stop and reflect on something in your life that is adding value to you. Before you start complaining about your rough day to your spouse, try to discover something that you can appreciate about them in that moment. If they're looking good, take a moment to compliment them and realize how lucky you are to have someone so beautiful in your life. If you can tell that they are sore from a hard day at work, thank them for being so dedicated to their job. Your desire to complain will dissipate as your new perspective draws you away from the destructive thought patterns of the past. *Damn, they look good.*

Another strategy for working appreciation into your relationship involves adding details to your gratitude and simply shifting your word choices in conversation. If you want your gratitude to be acknowledged on a deeper level, illuminate your words with clearer descriptions. *Why are you thankful?* For example, instead of simply thanking your partner for doing the dishes, give your compliment some color. An enhanced version might look like this: "That was so sweet of you to help with the clean-up tonight. I feel so lucky to have such a caring person in my life. Despite being tired after work, you still went above and beyond. Thank you."

Simple shifts in the way you approach your routine conversations is impactful. Try these simple approaches out for a few weeks and you will see the difference. Your discussions will begin to take on a kinder tone.

It's time to get creative

Now that you're starting to appreciate your partner a little more, let's discuss ways that you can begin to create excitement and freshness in your relationship. The seven-year itch has earned cliche status, but that itch won't stand a chance against your relationship when you add some creativity into the mix. Just like boredom is a symptom of lack of purpose, stagnancy in a relationship comes from a similar place. If you have lost sight of **why** you care so much for that person, and **why** you wanted the relationship in the first place, then refocus your attention on the ideas of appreciation that you wrote down earlier.

Developing renewed appreciation for your partner is the catalyst that will provide continuous motivation to stay creative in your love life. You deserve the best your relationship has to offer, and by implementing some innovative techniques, you will easily rekindle the love that was beginning to fade.

Whatever stage of the single, dating, or married life you're in, by adding unique twists and turns into your love playbook, you'll have a winning strategy. Being spontaneous and utilizing surprises when they least expect them will not only keep things fresh, but it will make the whole appreciating-each-other thing happen more naturally. The last thing you want to do is force romance, so the idea here is to seamlessly integrate creativity into your relationship.

I'd like you to think back to the section on passions. Hopefully you took the time to discuss and figure out which passions were beneficial for you and your relationship. If they had fun at that salsa dancing lesson with you, put that passion into your creative piggy bank for later withdrawal. Really start paying attention to what fascinates your partner and add those things to the piggy bank as well. As you discover more of your partner's interests, make sure to take note and figure out a way that you can get creative with that interest. Expressing interest in your partner's passions will illustrate just how important they are to you.

I've implemented creativity paired with the mutual passions we share in my relationship. For example:

- We went to a rock climbing gym together. We were both a little nervous about this since we'd never done anything like this before. We both have a mild fear of heights, but by encouraging each other and overcoming our fears, we conquered all three of the highest walls slowly but surely.

- I surprised her with a date night focused on reliving our first date together. I even called ahead to book the same table on the 2nd floor of the restaurant where we had our own private section. I took initiative by wearing the same nice button up shirt the first night we met. Instead of just another boring night out, this small gesture reflected that I wanted her to feel special and appreciated.

- I packed up our hiking bags and took her on a surprise trip. The beautiful trail was decorated with a scenic waterfall cascading down along the rocky walls nearby. Once at the top of the amazing trail, we had a photoshoot overlooking the waterfall. My handsome hound dog was the third wheel crashing our hike/date/adventure.

Come up with some of your own inspiring ideas. It's amazing just how far the little gestures can take you. By showing your partner that you are willing to put a little extra effort into creating a memorable time, they will feel valued and inspired to reciprocate. Your ideas don't need to be elaborate or complicated. Refer back to your list of passions and come up with some unique ideas.

Another important aspect of the creative challenge is to push your boundaries. Strive to find something that will be a new experience for both of you. As your relationship grows, so should the passions that you share. By constantly testing out new adventures in life, you'll be blown-away by how powerful these shared experiences can be. You may have to push through internal resistance or fear of change initially, but pay no mind to any thoughts holding you back from your creative inspirations. If that dance lesson seems like a horrifying idea, and images of stepping on your partners' toes flash through your mind, then it's time to schedule that dance class! That dance class that you dreaded so fiercely may lead to new friendships with other couples, close intimacy with your partner, and pride in finding out that you were a better dancer than you thought.

Earlier, I mentioned an interview with Will Smith that motivated me to pursue ideas that were intimidating. He speaks about the importance of *failing forward*. In a seemingly masochistic approach to life, he constantly seeks out new challenges that he is likely to fail at. This process builds a gradual resilience towards the things that we initially fear. He mentions his wife and how she ties into this lifestyle. She doesn't necessarily push herself in all of his specific endeavors, but she supports and encourages him throughout. Each of us must decide which areas we'd like to grow in. It's just an added bonus if your partner wants to go along for the ride. Remember to encourage them in whatever new outlet they are plugging into!

Even though our natural instincts have conditioned us to run when faced with fear, we must not heed that outdated programming. When was the last time your fight-or-flight response saved you from a bear? Probably never. In our comfortable and sterile modern world, our outdated human operating systems have yet to catch up. By understanding the usefulness of failing forward, we can embrace new experiences with open-arms and begin to undo the tendency to dwell in fear.

Think about anything you've ever feared. Chances are high that 99.9% of any fear based imagination has never come to fruition. This alone should stand as evidence that the creations of our minds are often out of alignment with our true capabilities. The sooner we begin taking action to face our fears and overcome the imaginary obstacles of our life, the sooner we can begin to experience the beautiful mysteries awaiting us on the other side. Are you going to listen to your fearful imagination, or are you going to take the courageous path of truth?

Romance is intentional

I hate breaking down *romance* into a timeline, but from my personal experience, the strategies for adding romance into your relationship need to be timed appropriately. Just like anything that was once exciting loses its luster if you over-engage in the action, I believe it's important to keep your surprises, surprising. If you lack creativity, and decide that you are only going to buy flowers once in a while for your loved one, then make sure you aren't giving them flowers every single week. Seriously, don't be that person. By timing your romantic tactics with unpredictability, you will enhance your efforts.

If you truly want to add value to your relationship, you can't settle for mediocre gestures to keep the spark fresh. If you find someone that is willing to tolerate you for an extended period of time, you owe it to them to make the life they have agreed to share with you an exciting one. Nobody wants to have a boring life with you. I don't care how well adjusted to the mind-numbing evenings you are, it's time to step it up and show your partner just how lucky they are to have you in their life.

Adding creativity into your love life will synergistically reinforce the new-found appreciation and gratitude mentalities you've cultivated for each other. By consistently acknowledging each other in thankfulness, challenging each other to try new things, and by keeping your relationship fresh through creative intention, you are one step closer to having the relationship you deserve. But remember, I *never* said this would be easy!

In the comedy series, "The League", the character Ruxin (played by Nick Kroll) details his innovative concept of the *Grand Gesture* when discussing a tip for creating a lasting marriage. Every few months, Ruxin emphasizes the importance of displaying his affection towards his wife through a *grand gesture.* While Ruxin may have selfish-motives and is simply doing the bare-minimum to keep his relationship intact, I have to admit that there is some validity to this plan. While I don't encourage this sort of relationship behavior for selfish motives, when a creative, unique, and carefully planned gesture is presented to your loved one, it serves as a valuable reminder of where your heart lies.

The key take away that I want to emphasize is the intentional focus on developing a selfless gesture. The *grand gestures* that you come up with should be tailored specifically to your partner and their love languages. By making regular and intentional action to reflect the feelings of your heart through a pronounced expression, you will prevent stagnation that is so common throughout long-term relationships.

I want you to take some time and brainstorm ideas that will light up your partner's life. Weed out any romantic ideas that are typical, repetitive, or just plain boring. Let your heart guide you throughout this exercise. If your heart is truly on fire for this other person, mediocre gestures will not be an accurate reflection of the passion that is within you. Do some research. Ask your friends for advice. Ask your partner about things that they are looking forward to. Just like you would take the appropriate amount of time to research a topic before writing an essay, understanding what truly speaks to your partners is equally important when designing thoughtful expressions for your partner.

This process should be as exciting for you as it is for them. These *grand gestures* are not only opportunities to express your love, but should enable growing closer together through new experiences while learning to appreciate each other more deeply. I want to reiterate - develop loving gestures that are exciting, genuine, and will inspire your partner to take an active participation in your love. Dig deep and discover just how much untapped passion is within you. The options for creating a deeper connection with your partner are limitless!

Hold on loosely, but don't let go

If you want your relationship to grow alongside new creative avenues, it's important to ease into these changes. If you're more of an extrovert, but your partner is inclined to prefer alone time, it's vital to remain conscientious of their needs with any new processes you hope to implement. Keep the creativity on a lighter note at first. Practicing patience with your partner throughout this process is imperative. If your partner is feeling pressured by you to grow, the kind-hearted intentions of yours can quickly back-fire.

In my current relationship, I made the mistake of trying to over-engage at times. I am a physically active individual who needs a daily dose of exercise to maintain a stable mental framework. My partner often needs to recharge her batteries after a long day at work, and I wasn't accurately gauging her susceptibility to my kind-hearted attempts to goad her into activities. What I had hoped would be simple encouragement to motivate her to exercise and enjoy nature with me, morphed into a perceived attack on her lifestyle. It wasn't that she was opposed to exercising with me, but she felt that I was pressuring her. She wanted to approach exercise at her own pace. I quickly realized that this was a sensitive subject for her, so I began to channel my creative efforts to bond with her in other ways. If she wasn't going to be my running buddy, that was completely fine. I found other ways to engage with her in a way that was less pushy yet accomplished the same end-goal of developing a closer bond. Instead, I discovered that she was interested in learning to cook and this outlet would achieve the same end result. We bought a new cookbook, learned some recipes, and started regularly cooking together.

Pacing your relationship growth by gradually inserting creativity relates to our previous topic on managing expectations. Remember, if your partner isn't as enthusiastic about certain passions as you are, no big deal. No matter what you hope to accomplish with creative relationship growth, it's important to remind yourself that your growth goals will never completely align with your loved one.

After you've deciphered the appropriate amount of creativity that you can add into your relationship, it will keep the staleness away, guaranteed. Continue to expect less, and simply be glad that they are in your life! If they do decide to join you on your next creative adventure, that's just an added bonus. Keep referring back to your thoughts of gratitude and why you are so glad that they're in your life the next time they tell you, "Honey, that sounds fun and all, but..."

Instead of feeling disheartened by potential creative rejections, use these instances to develop a deeper understanding of your partner. Don't become frustrated when you're told no. If the timing isn't right, recalibrate your efforts and try again later. Use rejections as opportunities to learn about new things that they might enjoy instead. By remaining receptive following rejection, you open the door for your partner to become inspired. Next time you're feeling inspired with a new date idea, perhaps pump your breaks and simply ask them what they would like to do. Letting them take control of the creative reigns will motivate them to join you in the pursuit of expanding your shared experiences.

What started as a rejection, will likely end in a collaborative idea. The end result: both of you feel valued and acknowledged throughout the process. Brainstorming ideas together has the added benefit of discovering new things about each other. Continue practicing patience throughout the process and find your creative balance. Adding creativity into your relationship should be a healthy and loving exchange, not a rushed process.

Shift your perspective and tailor your response

An important aspect of relationship growth is learning how to appropriately respond to disputes and troubles that are inevitable in your relationship. In any healthy relationship, it's important to be upfront and honest when you feel like a change needs to be made. Unfortunately, these valiant attempts to speak your mind and address your concerns often lead to heated arguments. But with a shift in your perspective and by learning how to tailor your response, fights in your relationship will be rare and easily overcome.

Couples today fight about everything and anything. Disputes erupt over dirty socks on the floor or what's for dinner that night. Anything that can be fought about, will be fought about- unless you decide to take the alternative route. If your relationship is plagued with battles, it's likely that you or your partner have been handling sensitive subjects incorrectly by making the problems personal. While minor disagreements may seem trivial, over time, these small battles create underlying tension in relationships. Arguments centered around serious topics like finances or finding day care for the kids are never solved through argument. Rather than solving the initial issue, it's likely that a new dispute forms. Arguing and fighting amplifies the problem while simultaneous creating mutual frustration until a resolution is impossible to achieve. That is no way to live. Instead, tension can be avoided by learning to master the art of negotiation. You may not be making a deal with a car salesman, but knowing how to reach peaceful resolutions through successful negotiation is a valuable tool for your relationship.

In the book "Getting to Yes: Negotiating Agreement Without Giving In" by Roger Fisher, I learned a powerful strategy for reaching a mutual solution without anyone feeling victimized. Creating distance between the issue at hand and the person with the grievance requires some careful word choices. Oftentimes, the problem presented has nothing to do with the person, but it becomes personal when their problem isn't acknowledged or is challenged defensively.

When confronted, focus entirely on the solution. Never focus on why that person caused the problem or why you aren't to blame. As soon as you become defensive or begin to blame, you wrap them up into the problem. This leads to personal attachment with that issue and can quickly spiral out of control into hurt feelings. When your efforts are focused on finding the solution, emotions are removed from the equation.

You have to be resilient and resist getting upset. Channel any initial knee-jerk anger or frustration into problem solving action. When someone is angry, it is tempting to be brought down to their level. It will take practice to avoid being sucked into that lower emotional frequency.

Continue focusing on actionable problem solving and you will remain detached from the problem. If you are successful at keeping the problem impersonal, your upset partner will learn to do the same. When the focus of your discussions transition from personal pain into problem solving action, negative emotions lose all traction.

If your partner approaches you with a problem that they're having, **listen and empathize** more than you speak. Try to understand exactly why they're upset before you attempt to give them your opinion of the proper solution. If it's a problem related to something that you're the cause of, try to offer realistic solutions to that problem without getting defensive. Also, maintaining a gentle tone of voice will reiterate that your realistic solution is being offered without sarcasm or superiority. You don't want providing a solution to be perceived as *knowing better than.* Empathize with their feelings by offering genuine condolences before giving excuses or blaming someone else. Even if you are entirely innocent, in that moment, let go of any pride you may have and be sensitive to the situation. Letting down your defenses can be a significant challenge if you have deeply-entrenched habits of pridefulness.

Forgive yourself if you temporarily falter and become defensive, but try and learn from those moments. You're only a victim if you decide to be, and by creating solutions instead of feeling attacked, a resolution is the likely outcome.

The simple act of practicing empathy goes a long way. But, that doesn't mean you should roll over and play dead every time you are confronted. You can stand your ground and assertively express your opinion without coming across as cruel or callous. If you listen with empathy and resist reacting defensively, yet, you still aren't able to resolve the issue, give each other some space. By giving your partner the breathing room that they need to reflect, oftentimes, the problem will resolve itself.

Another valuable tactic I've implemented when attempting to bring about a peaceful resolution is to write down grievances. Writing down your feelings can have a therapeutic effect and will make it easier to avoid a defensive or irrational knee-jerk reaction. This creates the space needed for a carefully constructed response.

Think of your grievance writing as a way to air your opinions through a rough draft. Review your initial thoughts, and edit them down to only the essential, solution oriented ideas. After a few minutes of writing, you may begin to realize how silly your anger was. When you see the issue from a different vantage point (the writer) you begin to see the anger for what it truly is- an unconscious, ego-based reaction that is centered in selfish desire rather than action oriented kindness. After a few practice writing sessions like this, you'll find that this process can eventually be skipped because you'll begin to respond with problem-solving kindness naturally.

Consider your tone of voice. Nobody likes to be talked down to, belittled, or intimidated. When someone is upset, they are already feeling violated or vulnerable, and responding with a negative or judgemental tone will only add fuel to the flames. Do your best to remain calm and gentle with your words. This is the love of your life you are speaking with, so they deserve to be treated as such. If the tone you're using wouldn't be appropriate when speaking to a stranger or a child then don't use that tone with your partner. It's really not that hard to speak with courteous gentleness, but it does take practice if you have a habit of reacting with snippy, irritated, or grumpy retorts. This goes for those plaintive sighs as well. Responding with a kinder tone sets the mood for how the rest of the conversation will play out.

Take notice of your body language and posturing. Subtle changes in the way you carry yourself can ease tension during any confrontation. Aggressive gestures send a message that you are closed off and uninterested; open postures and soft facial expressions convey that you are ready to listen and consider their needs without judgement. If you're hoping to reach a resolution, do your best to avoid body language such as: crossed arms or legs, yawning, tight lipped grimaces, balled fists, or eye-rolls/lack of eye contact.

There are countless other subtleties, but begin to pay attention to the way people in your life carry themselves. When one of your friends or co-workers gets upset, try to decode their body language; take note of their posturing when they are feeling irritated, confident, or happy. Some compassionate gestures and ideas include: smiling and soft facial expressions, opening your stance (uncross arms and legs), leaning in (show you are listening and interested) or leaning back (relaxed postures convey openness and calmness). As you become more adept in your body language awareness, you can mimic the successful gestures you see and apply them towards your daily interactions.

By remaining open to grievances with compassionate and gentle responses, your chances of reaching a peaceful solution multiply. Separate the person from the problem; develop an action plan to solve that problem without making it personal. Practice empathy by considering their point of view from their shoes. Continue to keep your tone of voice and body language in check. You will begin to see a shift in your relationship. These subtle changes have lasting effects that will gradually turn consistent arguments into happy endings.

If you consistently practice renewed gentleness towards your partners' issues yet you find grievances continue to materialize, there is a good chance that an underlying concern isn't being addressed. You'll be able to detect these subtle frustrations if you have adequately addressed the problem at hand but feel that your partner is still dissatisfied. This can occur when you have successfully treated the problems' symptom, rather than the deeper emotional issue at hand. You must become a master emotional investigator. I emphasized **listening** earlier because by carefully considering the intent beneath their concerns, the fundamental cause of their frustrations will become more apparent.

Arguments can actually be catalysts for growth in your relationship. Once you have discovered the true source of the dispute, begin to discuss solutions and create a plan to prevent this problem from recurring. Continue to keep the problem separate from the person. Remember, the key is to maintain an open and calm demeanor so that your partner will be able to speak honestly.

You want to create a safe space for them. If you can successfully transform the anger of the current situation into an honest dialogue, you will learn new things about your partner instead of battling each other. This can be a difficult transformation, but once you put your new listening and empathy skills to work, you'll find that disagreements strengthen rather than damage your relationship in the long-run. Trust is established, closeness emerges, and fights will begin to seem trivial because the love that you share consistently overcomes.

Learning to be present

"So the single most vital step on your journey toward enlightenment is this: Learn to disidentify from your mind." -Eckhart Tolle

I am a fan of the book "A New Earth" by Eckhart Tolle. It's a valuable resource for learning how to effectively manage problems you encounter within your relationship. The author discusses how the problems we have in life are simply extensions of our mind's creation. All problems that arise in our lives are a result of unfulfilled, and often, unrealistic expectations that are fueled by the false narrative our minds create.

When we let go of the illusion that our lives should go the way that we think they should go, life becomes much more peaceful. The more we practice distancing ourselves from the impossible-to-satisfy needs of our minds, the more readily joy will fill our moments. If you can understand this concept, the next time you are frustrated with your partner about something they did or didn't do, anger will never develop and the problem will dissolve before it reaches your lips.

Most of our relationship woes can be traced to something

from the past or the future. Think about the last time your partner became upset about something. Let's say they were mad because you left your muddy shoes in the kitchen. Were either of your lives negatively impacted? Yes, the floor is dirty. Yes, you didn't listen to their previous request of leaving your shoes outside. But, **no**, your existence was not damaged, destroyed, or impacted in any meaningful way. This is the case with all of our problems. Our egos like to take control and manufacture false pain. The ego is needy and wants your attention. The ego will use any tool at its disposal to get that attention, even if that means creating *illusory pain* through anger or frustration. Let's look closely at the muddy shoe scenario and discover how this problem is simply a manufactured illusion.

The moment of anger over the muddy shoes was spent in a low-frequency state of anger. In reality, nothing really happened to your upset partner. But, their mind categorized this superficial muddy-mess as a personal attack. Anger can only exist while in a semi-conscious state. The mind has taken control and says, "He never listens or appreciates how hard I work to keep this house clean!" At the root of this thought, you can see that the mind has created an expectation for a clean floor. As you know, it is **impossible** to satisfy this expectation. Messes will always happen, and continue to happen long after you are dead. The creations of our minds come up with impossibilities like this every single day. It is imperative that we learn to ignore these thoughts that are rooted in false expectations. Learn to engage **only** with the thoughts that are solution-oriented, loving, or based in reality and you will quickly discover how often our minds try to deceive us.

Instead of reacting to the dirty floor with anger, a more present approach to the situation would have sufficed. If you can achieve the same end result (a clean floor) without anger, then what purpose does the anger serve? Becoming upset did not solve the problem. Cleaning up the floor and reminding your partner to remove their shoes were the only necessary steps. Apply this example to other *problems* you face within your relationship and you will begin to see that every situation can be handled without anger.

Instead of just cleaning up the muddy shoes and asking your partner to avoid doing that in the future, an argument starts that could have been easily avoided. Every time you face a problem like this, bring an active awareness to what is currently happening. Unless your life is presently endangered, it's probably not worth getting all fired up about. When you learn to transition from the "I'm the victim" mindset to the "how can I fix this right now" mindset, resolutions that were once a distant hope are rapidly attained.

While this sounds good in theory, it truly is quite simple to make this transition. We have been conditioned to latch onto the thoughts of the problems we have in life. When we listen to and believe every thought that crosses our minds, we become slaves to the machinations of the mind. We are living as servants to our thoughts. The only way to break free from this servitude is to recognize that our minds are simply tools to be used for our continual growth. When we ignore the manipulative thoughts that frequent our mind-space, and focus only on thoughts that are practical and useful, our precious mental energy transforms into a force for creative solutions rather than senseless anger.

This may seem like an impossible task because it's likely that your mind has called the shots throughout your life. If you are ready to take back control of your life and your relationship, learning to live in the moment and to ignore your impossible-to-satisfy ego is an important step. We are all on different paths in life, and perhaps you may not be ready or willing to consider this change quite yet, but give it a chance. Worst case scenario: nothing changes. Best case scenario: You find a richer contentment in life and share that contentment with the ones you love.

I'd like you to sit quietly for a few minutes and pay attention to your thoughts. Imagine that you are standing in an open field. When you look up into the sky, imagine that each cloud passing by is a thought.

In this example, you are separate from your thoughts. You are on the ground, the clouds are floating by, and there is space between you and the clouds.

Just watch the clouds floating by.

These are your thoughts.

They are not you.

Now take a few moments to become aware of your breath. Feel the cool air as it passes through your nostrils and into your throat. Feel your chest as it gently fills with air. Pay attention to the sensation of air passing over your lips as you exhale.

Keep your attention focused on your breathing.

While continuing to focus on your breathing, you will find that more clouds begin to cross your minds' eye. The clouds keep floating along whether you like it or not, because that is the nature of the mind. The mind continuously creates new clouds, and your ego constantly vies for your attention.

Understand this:

The ego **cannot** survive without you.

You **can** survive without the ego.

Instead of latching onto the first cloud that crosses your mind, ignore that cloud. Do not let that cloud take control of your attention, and simply let it float on by. Bring your attention back to your breathing. You are still sitting quietly on the ground below. It is hard to ignore the clouds. You want to latch. Your thoughts are not in control.

Keep watching the clouds.

Do not give them your attention.

Focus on the sensations of your breath.

Continue imagining that your thoughts are clouds passing by. You are on the ground below, watching them. As they continue to come and go, you ignore them. You are separate from your thoughts. You still exist, regardless of whether or not you give those thoughts the attention they crave. Breathe. Feel the air passing through your nostrils as you breathe in. Notice the sensations in your mouth, throat and lungs as your lungs move the air in and out. Keep your focus on your breath. The clouds keep passing by. Pay them no attention.

You have a thought that you need to take the dog outside, and worry that if you don't hurry the dog will pee on the new rug. Let that thought go by while you continue to breathe. Focus on the sensations. As you continue to watch the clouds float by and listen to your breathing, a deep inner peace begins to replace any tension or worries that were present. **You are not your thoughts.** Your ego is like a needy friend needing constant reassurance that it is making the right choices. Your mind is simply a tool to use for connecting with the world around you and for solving problems, not something that should dictate your life.

By discovering the truth that your true self is separate from your thoughts, you can begin to take back control of your life and become more present in your relationship. When you are living in a state of conscious awareness of the present moment; disengaging from the lies that your mind creates on a regular basis, you are available to give your partner the very best of you. When you are lost in a spiral of thoughts that serve no purpose, you are detached from the wonderful life you have right in front of your eyes. This understanding takes a willingness to change. It will take dedicated and conscious effort because time and time again your mind will try to suck you back into the void of self-defeating thoughts of worries and fears.

I recommend you come up with a way to remind yourself to come back to the present moment in some way. It can be anything from a sticky note on your desk or the word **NOW** scrawled on your hand in pen. Simply come up with a way to remind yourself to come back to now. If you feel that remaining in the present moment and only focusing on the reality that is directly in front of your eyes is a challenge, make your reminders more prominent. Set a daily reminder on your phone that sends you alerts throughout the day. The alert can simply read: Focus on your breathing right now.

My present practice is simple. I pay attention to my feet. The feeling of my socks and shoes, the pressure of the ground pressing into me, or any muscle soreness or pain I may have. Throughout the day, I regularly re-center myself by bringing my attention back to the sensations of my feet. By shifting my attention to physical sensations, this serves as a reminder to be aware of what is currently happening. My thoughts want to take me to a fear or worry for tomorrow that **doesn't** exist. The physical sensations I'm currently having **do** exist. This physical sensation is simply acting as a reminder to be aware of now.

I appreciate the symbolic focus that our feet have in connection with the earth, but feel free to decide for yourself what your go-to re-centering focus will be. It can be anything that brings you back to now. Keep it simple. Any time you become aware that your mind is spiraling out of control, become aware of the centering action you've chosen. This will take significant practice, and at the beginning, you may not even be aware that you are lost in your thoughts. You have grabbed onto a passing cloud. You have forgotten that you are still existing on the ground below.

I have a natural propensity to worry. So, this process of overcoming my ego has been an ongoing battle. My mind is often successful and pulls me down the path of self-defeating thoughts. But, the more I practice paying attention to the present moment, the more readily I reach a state of calm awareness. Once you make your present-trigger a habit, it will become easier and easier to get out of your head and to live in a peaceful state centered in reality. In time, your defeating thoughts lose their power over you. Your mind simply becomes a tool for problem solving that works in tandem with your true self to create consistent inner-peace. If you can understand this simple concept, you will begin to operate on a higher-frequency in all areas of your life.

By living in a state of presence, a deeper love exists

If you decide that separation for your old patterns is too much of a stretch, no big deal. We have to decide for ourselves which ideas we choose to implement into our lives. Even if you find that you and your ego want to remain intertwined indefinitely, hopefully you will start giving less credibility to the unrealistic expectations created by your ego. It is a complicated process to let go of a life-long system of beliefs regarding *who* you are.

By learning that our minds aren't in control, and understanding that our true selves remain in a constant state of judgement-free peace, we will become free. This is an ongoing learning process and will require long-term focused commitment. For many people, this is a new concept and requires unlearning years and years of cognitive deceit. The end result if you are successful: a renewed perspective in life that empowers you while simultaneously opening your heart and mind to the many exciting opportunities you have overlooked thus far. My relationship has shifted from the ego asking, "How can they please me?" to my true-self knowing that, "I am so happy to have them in my life right **now**."

The topics we've discussed so far are centered on the principle of remaining present and aware of your current situation. The ability to live in the present moment allows for a deeper connection in your relationship. I challenge you to spend five intentional minutes today with your partner. These five minutes should be dedicated to connecting with them. Instead of your usual conversation, think of this as a shared meditation. I recommend that you sit facing them, perhaps hold each-others' hands, and proceed to share these minutes of calmness together.

Try to leave your worries about the past and the future behind. This time is for you and your partner. During this time, don't discuss finances, the chores you have to do, or what someone said to you at work. All of these thoughts take you away from **now**. Do not let your mind steal this time away from you. This time is for you and your partner to simply exist together and practice awareness for each other. It's only five minutes today, but the rewards will pay you in dividends throughout the course of your relationship.

As you initiate this process with your partner, come up with some simple triggers to remind each other to remain in the moment. For example, as you're holding hands, you can gently squeeze each other with each exhaled breath. During your initial sessions together, assisting each other with consistent reminders to stay focused on the moment is invaluable. This process may be more difficult than you imagine, but if you have the desire to connect deeply with your partner on a spiritual level, continue practicing meditative breathing sessions together. In time, reaching a state of inner calm will come more readily as you learn to unwind from the trappings of your minds. The benefits from this practice include improved health, decreased stress, and a unique closeness to your partner.

Schedule present moments with your partner

In our fast-paced world, it is easy to be swept away with the turmoil. By learning to share scheduled, present moments in your relationship, you become a source of renewal for each other. The more regularly you share these moments together, the more powerful the effect becomes. Persistent arguments will become a thing of the past. As you discover how irrelevant your disputes were, you will learn to laugh at the things you used to fight about. When you are completely connected with each other in calm awareness, words will not be able to describe the powerful depth of love that emerges.

That's why it's important to set a schedule for this. We have to resist the daily trappings of our modern world. If we aren't intentional with this relationship growth, it can easily be displaced with other obligations. Add this to your list of expectations for your relationship, and explain to your partner why this is important to you. Even if your partner is skeptical about this shared meditation, ask that they at least try it once or twice. If they aren't on board to begin with, they may be pleasantly surprised by the experience. There is magic in the present moment, and when that experience is shared, the experience becomes even more profound. Give it a try. It only takes five minutes. Make this a regular addition to your relationship once you have a few trial runs under your belt.

Surround yourself with supportive influences

Creating an environment that encourages your growth is essential to your long-term relationship health. Developing your passions, practicing gratefulness, and becoming more aware of your present moment will assist you in this next step of cultivating an environment that encourages your growth. While each of the areas of growth we've covered are important, becoming highly selective of the influences that you choose to surround yourself with will reinforce those new skill sets.

Transitioning from a lifestyle filled with toxic influences into a lifestyle filled with supportive influences will take courage. Influences that sap our energy are multi-faceted and seemingly omnipresent. I could list a million different toxic forces in the world, but here are a few obvious culprits that you may be familiar with:

News: Most of the information that we receive is not relevant to our current life. Unless you are watching the weather channel, or your job directly relates to the news, you would likely be better off without this source of relentless fear creation. Ask yourself, does the information that you receive from the news really add value to your life? If anything you're missing is **that important**, you'll hear about it from your friends and family.

Family, Friends, Co-Workers: Carefully consider all of your closest relationships. Are these people contributing to your life in a meaningful way? Truthfully answering this question is vital to your mental well-being and relationship success. There are many aspects of life that you cannot control, but choosing whom you are willing to spend time with **is** something that you can control. Even if it's a work colleague who was cast upon your shared office space, there is always a way to create distance. Once you have carefully weighed the relationships in your life, decide which ones are in alignment with your long-term goals. This may seem callous, but it is imperative that you muster the courage to remove toxic relationships whenever possible. Every relationship has pros and cons, and deciding which course of action is appropriate can be a complicated process. Deciding to end a relationship can be a painful process but is often necessary.

Addictions: If you struggle with drugs or alcohol, take

steps to remove these influences in your life. If you struggle with gambling or online-shopping, take steps to remove the access to those vices. Refer back to the section on rewiring your habits. Sometimes, addictions have a way of subconsciously intertwining with our lives. The cliche, "The first step on the road to recovery is recognizing that you have a problem," is relevant here.

"The journey of a thousand miles begins with a single step." -Lao Tzu

To discover any potential addictions in your life that are holding you back, ask yourself, "Could I easily walk away from this influence in my life?" For example, if you think you're not an alcoholic, but your natural response to stress is to automatically reach for a glass of wine, then you may have an underlying addiction that you haven't acknowledged. Once you identify aspects of your life that you'd be better off without, take action to change or remove these influences. Don't listen to the hundreds of different reasons why you can't live without that influence. Focus on the solution. How much more free time, cash, and mental-clarity would you bring to your relationship without that influence?

Change for the better

In any situation, we have three choices: accept it, change it, or remove yourself from it. It's important to develop your own criteria for what you are willing to tolerate. For starters, think about some of the influences in your life that are creating tension. Many of the influences that we accept could be easily changed for the better or removed altogether. I am an advocate for positive change and acceptance, but have learned to remove toxicity like a surgeon.

I strive to apply the first two choices, acceptance and change, prior to removing the majority of influences in my life. Some may perceive this propensity to see the best in people or situations as a weakness, but I believe that everyone deserves acceptance and a chance to change for the better. There are obvious exceptions to this acceptance and hope for change, and only you can ultimately decide what you are willing to put up with or sacrifice. Sometimes, certain influences aren't worth tolerating for more than a second, and can be immediately cut-out. It is up to you to develop and decide which environmental factors are most conducive to your well-being and love-life.

Deciding which influences in your life belong, versus those that don't, can be a lengthy pursuit. A specific friend comes to mind because he was motivated, fun to be around, and had a fresh perspective for the world. Throughout the span of our friendship, we experienced many unique adventures and shared some good times. But ultimately, this friendship wasn't in alignment with my long-term goals for a number of reasons.

My kind-hearted nature resisted the instinctual warning signs. I knew deep down that something about our friendship needed to change. As we grew closer in our friendship, I realized that this person was very self-serving and was solely focused on temporary pleasures. Since I'm the type of person that wants to fix something before I throw it away, I made it clear how I was feeling in the hopes of inspiring change. I felt that I was being used as a party supplier, wing-man, and only someone to joke around with. Whenever I tried to address how I was feeling or asked a favor of him, he would laugh the topic off and proceed to serve himself. My efforts to share meaningful topics and express my feelings were brushed under the rug and belittled.

Other toxic aspects of the relationship began to emerge. At the beginning, he would have only a drink or two. But his drug and alcohol usage began to significantly increase. I had clearly explained earlier in the friendship that I was a recovering alcoholic, and to please stop requesting that I imbibe with him. My requests were simple, yet they were consistently ignored. This became more apparent as the one-sided nature of this relationship progressed. I was naively paying for many things, and was always met with an intricate excuse whenever the bill was passed his way. At this point, I became hyper-aware of just how poor our relationship had become. The close friendship that we had originally shared was now a source of toxicity in my life.

I knew that his trajectory was diverging from any hope for a healthy relationship. I originally accepted some of his behaviors because we were having fun. But the fun was over, and I was left feeling used and deceived. Despite my efforts to change this friendship into a mutually beneficial relationship, he was unwilling to work with me. I ultimately removed myself from the relationship entirely.

It was a stressful conversation when I finally worked up the courage to confront him. He was perplexed, frustrated and said that I was being cruel. But through expressing these sentiments, I knew that he was trying to manipulate me. When trying to remove a toxic relationship from your life, a common tactic employed by the abuser is gas-lighting. By flipping the blame onto your shoulders, saying "You don't care about this friendship, you're being so selfish!" the enticing guilt trip can lure you into their trap.

Instead of escaping from the poisonous relationship, you are tricked into apologizing and asking them for forgiveness! This is common among domestic assault cases in which the abused partner remains in the relationship because they have been duped into believing that they are the reason for the violence. If the abuser is exceptionally adept with deception, a victim might even become convinced that they are delusional and were never assaulted in the first place. It was all in their imagination.

Finding the courage to remove toxic situations like this from your life can be a daunting task. The life of a hoarder is an analogy that comes to mind when removing toxic baggage from our lives. I've watched a few episodes of the show, "Hoarders," and noticed a similar theme throughout. Every person featured in the show has developed a crippling attachment to the clutter in their life. This is exactly the same as many of the toxic influences present in our lives.

The process of removing all of the garbage from within their homes is a highly controversial transition for many of these individuals. The reasons behind their attachment to these things may differ, but ultimately, they are based on an unrealistic expectation. The objects being hoarded are rationalized as essential or important for sentimental reasons. This relates to our relationship baggage, because oftentimes, we rationalize unhealthy aspects of our relationships as essential. The garbage needs to be taken out. It doesn't matter how important you think that trash is. If the accumulated garbage in your life isn't directly useful or relevant to your daily life, get rid of it!

I had to remove several toxic friendships before I could successfully maintain a sober and love-filled life. I would start making steps towards recovery, only to be lured back into old patterns with tempting promises of excitement and a night to remember. Many of the so-called friends that I surrounded myself with were genuinely kind people. But, the road to hell is paved with kind intention. None of these people meant to encourage my toxic behaviors. However, the inevitable outcome of spending time with these people created lifestyle habits that were detrimental. When virulent behavior becomes commonplace in social gatherings, other healthier activities are not taken into consideration.

When toxicity pervades your relationship sphere, this creates a distorted *fish bowl effect.* Just like the fish isn't aware of the fact that they are immersed, it can be difficult to see the true nature of your current toxic situation when you are in its grasps. I was a victim of this effect throughout the majority of my twenties. Due to poor choices and pleasure seeking, I quickly found myself surrounded with like-minded individuals. The sole purpose of our social gatherings was to perpetuate self-serving behaviors. If drugs or alcohol weren't involved, we wouldn't have a reason to gather. This created a social pattern that encouraged poor choices, and resisted any positive forces that deviated from the "fun."

It wasn't until I had removed myself from that sludge-filled fish bowl that I finally began to see things with a clearer perspective. The catalyst for change was a deep-longing within me to find joy in life. I was sick and tired of being sick and tired. I had found my strong reason. This reason was the catalyst that motivated me to move across the country and start a new life in the mountains. Since I was unwilling to accept my current situation, and changing the lifestyle of my friends was not an option, the only choice I felt that I had left was to remove myself. Of course, I could have abandoned the poisonous influences and started a new life right then and there, but I wasn't yet mentally tough enough to go cold turkey on the toxicity. In this instance, removing the toxic influence by removing myself was the key.

I had discovered my reason (I wanted to find joy in life), and the motivation to continue on this journey has persisted since. I hope that you can find a strong enough reason for yourself. Focusing on what you're grateful for will help to reinforce this reason. The reason for why you want a healthy relationship needs to be in the back of your mind at all times. Do not let your thoughts and worries prevent you from making the changes that you need.

Once you remove certain poisonous influences from your life, your relationship will greatly benefit. If you have a friend that is constantly bad mouthing your boyfriend when you know it is undeserved, tread with caution. Judge-mental whisperings can undermine your relationship. However, an exception should be made with friends that are giving you hard to hear advice. If that friend has previously provided you with trustworthy and valuable feedback, then that constructive criticism should be taken into consideration.

The truth hurts, and perhaps your boyfriend really does suck. If you have a friend that has always been truthful with you and encourages your relationship, you will be inspired to bring that positive energy into your relationship. Choose to remain in contact with the encouraging friend, and distance yourself from the trash-talker. Really listen to the people in your life, evaluate their information for truthfulness, and decide for yourself whose advice is reliable. Do the people in your life support your **reason?**

Have courage and remove toxicity

Remain resolute once you have decided which influences need to go. Put them in writing. If your gut is telling you something is bringing you down, don't listen to the excuses for why that influence is essential. If it's consistently stealing your joy in any way, you have no time for it. If it doesn't align with your life and relationship goals, it is slowing you down.

Now that you know what needs to change in your life, it's time to take the necessary action. Make a list of all of the detrimental influences in your life. I recommend starting your list with the most gripping influences first. Narrow the influence down to a specific idea. The more specific the idea, the more direct your action will be. Whenever I want to tackle a set of goals, I start with the most difficult task first. Next to each of these items, make another column labeled: Accept, Change, Remove. Now, make a third column titled: Action Steps.

Bad Influence	Accept, Change, Remove	Action Steps
Nicotine	Change	Replace smoking routine with exercise
Angry friend	Remove	Tell them how I feel and cease to contact
Staying up too late	Accept	None, I choose to stay up late sometimes
Anger over dishes	Change	Talk about ways that we can compromise and split up chores

If you live your life trying to please others, you will limit your potential. In order to truly be of service to others in your life, you have to put yourself first. It may seem like backwards logic, but being a little selfish is truly selfless when focusing on the bigger picture. You are able to live up to your full potential once you have spent the appropriate amount of effort to serve yourself. The seemingly selfish, yet rich man, is a prime example. Someone might call the business tycoon selfish for being so greedy. But following that business tycoons' ascension to riches, perhaps he then donates millions of dollars to a charity that aids impoverished communities. The person who called that business tycoon selfish might be living a life that they consider to be less selfish. They occasionally volunteer. They recycle and conserve water. They judge the rich man, yet are only able to donate ten dollars to that same charity. In this case, the rich man is far from selfish, but the naive onlooker is unaware of the kind hearted intention hidden beneath the self-serving appearances.

Help others by helping yourself first! Toxic influences will relentlessly try to derail your self-growth. Don't let them! Keep taking action every day to create the life you and your partner deserve.

As you successfully transition away from influences that were weighing you down, positive influences will be drawn to you. Misery loves company, and so does kindness. Instead of spending time with a group of gossipers, ask your encouraging friend to introduce you to other people that live in alignment with your new path. Any negative influence that you successfully remove from your life will be replaced with its polar opposite as your discernment improves. All of these replaced influences will directly manifest into a healthier you and a healthier relationship.

Motivation comes during the practice in action, not before. When I think about training for a half-marathon, I have discouraging thoughts. Instead of listening to those thoughts, I ease into the training by creating a simple schedule. This alleviates the perceived difficulty by designing a filtered version. Even though the mileage is exactly the same, I have successfully tamed my defeating thoughts by providing a less painful option.

Once I have the training schedule down on paper, broken into simple segments, the task is less intimidating. Instead of thinking, "Holy goodness. Running 40 miles a week is insanity!" I look at the schedule and think, "I can easily run six miles today. It'll only take an hour!" Even that six miles might seem like a lot for one day, so I break it down even further. I tell myself, "I'll just do a practice mile and see how I feel." After running that first mile, the defeating thoughts transition into, "That was easy, let's keep going." Before I know it, I've completed the six miles and feel a sense of pride.

Try this "easing into it" approach with the influences

you are trying to replace. Instead of looking at the necessary changes from a scary cliff side, compartmentalize the changes taking place into smaller, bite size increments. If you have a cruel friend, but you feel obligated to be in their life, start by gradually spending less time with them. As you slowly back away from that relationship, you will begin to notice that it wasn't as stressful as you'd imagined. Begin to create distance in that relationship. The benefits will become more obvious. You will begin to see the relationship for what it was. This process will get easier and easier as your courage and self-worth increases.

Laughter is the best medicine

Keep things light-hearted in your love life! Life is only as serious as you make it. If you're treating your love life like a chemistry equation, it's bound for blandness. I want to have fun in my relationship. I want my face to hurt from smiling so hard. I want to feel that deep connection that comes from sharing moments of blissful laughter. I want you to have that.

Think about a first date you had with someone that you really clicked with. You could be yourself; you felt completely comfortable and were honest about the details of your life. You wanted to show that person how much excitement and value you could add to their life. You didn't focus on the problems in your life; you presented your best self and brought a smile to their face. Why should that change. Remember Bill and his 60- year relationship success advice from earlier? *Treat your partner like you did on day one.* Of course issues will arise along your relationship journey, but these issues will diminish if you can remember the initial reasons you fell in love. By reliving those blissful first experiences together, you're liable to repeat those successful moments later on.

Falling out of love is a myth. It is a failure to remember why you were initially so attracted to that person. Instead of choosing to focus on why you are grateful for that person, you focus on how they aren't meeting your expectations. You used to laugh together. You used to share your interesting life experiences with a smile on your face. You told them about the things you found beautiful and the hobbies that lit your fire. Hold those moments you shared together in your heart, and your love will grow.

When you keep humor at the forefront of your relationship, you refresh your relationship. If your relationship feels like it's in a rut, think about some of the earlier moments of joy that you shared. Go and look up some jokes or find some hilarious cat videos to share. Think about some of the passions and creative ideas you came up with earlier to inspire some smiles in your relationship. Only you know the secret to unlocking that charming smile of theirs!

Get over yourself and that calloused world-view. If you have a pessimistic outlook, and you feel like implementing humor into your relationship is hopeless, then consider this. You have two options: You can either be a pessimist or an optimist. If you are a pessimist, and all of your worries come to fruition, then you were right. So what? You spent your life worrying and fretting, yet your outlook didn't change the result. If you are an optimist, and your positive outlook doesn't work out like you had hoped, at least you will have lived joyfully. It doesn't make sense to live any other way! View all aspects of your relationship with optimism rather than pessimism. I know I'd rather be laughing instead of arguing.

I challenge you to make your partner laugh today. As a matter of fact, I dare you! Do they like cheesy jokes, or is sarcasm more their style? Figure out how to get under their skin and yank that smile out of them if you have to! When you regularly smile with each other, love is so much easier.

Wife: "How would you describe me?"   Husband: "ABCDEFGHIJK."

Wife: "What does that mean?"

Husband: "Adorable, beautiful, cute, delightful, elegant, fashionable, gorgeous, and hot."

Wife: "Aw, thank you, but what about IJK?"

Husband: "I'm just kidding!"

Solutions for lacking intimacy

Just like we all need love, we all need physical touch. I have yet to meet someone that would disagree! The benefits of intimate physical contact are limitless. The appropriate amount that you or your partner desire may differ, but it is imperative that you learn their preferences and begin to involve intimacy. Psychologists, philosophers, and scientists all have differing perspectives on the subject, but all would agree that physical connections are necessary for a healthy life. Whether the physical and emotional response resulting from touch is chemical or spiritual in nature, it doesn't matter to me. What matters is that we strive to keep a healthy dose of physical touch in our lives!

Feeling under-prescribed in the intimacy department? I'm here to help you get that dosage right. Oftentimes, lack of physical intimacy isn't a result of poor performance in the bedroom (although this might be the case), but rather a deficiency in the emotional department. If you feel like you've been cut off from the regular cuddle sessions you used to share, think about what other aspects of your relationship you may be neglecting. Have you been practicing gratitude, listening to their frustrations, and helping around the house?

The solution to your bedroom woes may become obvious once you think about the chores you've been putting off.

"Want to avoid conflict? Well, she won't yell at you while you're folding the laundry." -L.S.

Are you taking action to focus on your health and appearance? I would never encourage exercise or dressing nicely for purely vain or superficial reasons. When you think about how you can better serve your partner, don't you want to be healthy and attractive? By making a diligent effort to stay in shape, you will be an addition to you and your partner's well-being. I could list a thousand reasons why regularly exercising has benefited my relationship, but here are a few examples:

- More energy to help with chores around the house
- More stamina in the bedroom (round two anyone?)
- Indirectly encourages healthy habits in partners' life (when she sees me going for a run, she is inspired to do a yoga session)
- Remaining attractive to partner
- Sick less (less dependence on each other)
- Sharpened mind (clearer communication; improved listening)

If you are completely honest with yourself, having a partner that you feel attracted to is important. Ultimately, looks will fade, and the emotional connection is more important, but that doesn't discount the truth of the matter. We are sexual beings, and if we deny our instinctual urges based on physical attraction, we are denying ourselves one of life's greatest pleasures and risk distancing ourselves from our partners.

By taking the time to accentuate our appearance, the result is a win-win situation. Self-care increases feelings of self-worth and confidence. This self-worth and confidence will transfer into your love life. If you feel better about yourself, you will naturally bring a more positive energy into your love life. Remember the self-serving rich man from before? This scenario applies here. Out of a gratefulness and respect for your life and everything in it, physical self-care is vital.

If your partner's love language is *words of affirmation*, imagine how impactful your affirmation will be following their work-out routine. They were beaming after their plyometric session, and are met with grateful acknowledgment when you say, "I'm so proud of you for pushing yourself like that." In this case, affirmative acknowledgment leads to more passion in the bedroom because your partner feels valued and encouraged. But don't be encouraging towards your partner simply for the reward. The pleasure of intimacy is the natural bonus that manifests from treating your partner with the respect and compassion they deserve.

Begin by taking full account of your current physical fitness level. Decide on a target weight or strength level you'd like to reach. When creating a plan to improve your fitness, it's important to be specific. If you don't have a clearly defined goal, it's easy to come up with excuses for taking a day off and you will stray from your original plan. I recommend starting with easily attainable goals such as losing 10 pounds or being able to lift slightly heavier weights. If you keep the target simple during the initial phase, making exercise a part of your life will flow naturally. Just like the habit loop we discussed earlier, rewiring your daily routines to enhance your fitness is a challenge worth overcoming for you and your partner.

Remember why you want a successful love life and think back to some of your passions. The more reasons you can come up with to stay on track and to reach that *happy-ever-*

after, the more likely you'll stay on track to your goals. If you are the type of person that likes to plan ahead and organize everything, writing down your work-out routine may be the best solution. If you are the type of person that just goes with the flow and doesn't like to plan more than five minutes in advance, then your reason for reaching your goals will have to be hard-wired into your daily mental planning. Look back at your list of passions and pick an idea that you can harness into a daily motivation mantra.

When I am tired from a long day at work and the couch lures me into wasting away the day, I counteract these temptations with a few hard-wired strategies. First, I think about a long term goal of becoming a competitive disc-golfer. I visualize myself lining up the perfect throw and what it would take to have that competitive edge. I visualize how my body turns in perfect harmony as the ideal shot is released and lands gently next to the basket. I need to be in top shape in order to remain consistent. With a renewed fire in my heart, I tie up my tennis shoes and spring through the door with my head held high.

With the newfound confidence and energy you'll have from improved fitness, take note of how these changes reflect in your relationship. If you were doing everything else right before but your gut was bursting through your way-too-tight shirt, it's possible that your elevated fitness will reignite the spark in your partner's eye. There really is no downside to improving your health other than the temporary discomfort from exercise and a stricter diet. Are you ready to fight for your health?

Think outside of the bedroom

It's possible that all of your emotional bases are covered, yet the intimacy is still missing. Hopefully by now, you've started implementing ideas from previous chapters into your relationship. These steps are essential for building the solid foundation in which intimacy can flourish. There are a number of reasons why the bedroom excitement might be fading, so don't be discouraged if your attempts to improve your relationship haven't transitioned into more intimacy. Be patient. Continue working on the areas of weakness within your relationship and you **will** see results.

"Do not relegate sex to a mechanical act. Celebrate it as a continuum of attraction between you and your partner." -Unknown

Getting creative with intimacy doesn't begin in the bedroom. Start slipping compliments and affection into your daily interactions. My partner's main love language, physical touch, is affirmed regularly throughout the day with genuine hugs, hand holding, and massage. The ten second hug or five-minute massage is a great way to remind my partner that they are high on my list of priorities. Even if your partners' primary love language differs, taking the time to show how much you care with genuine affection can go a long way. With the time that you set aside for your partner today, take action to add compassionate touch and affirmation into the mix.

Routines can be helpful when reshaping habits, but routines can also lead to dullness in your sex life. A routine love life sounds to me like monotony with a hint of soul numbing. You can avoid that horrific scenario by adding creative and kinky diversity into your love life. Experimenting with different techniques is a fantastic way to find pleasure in exploring each other. Just like you had to step outside of your comfort zone while discovering new passions, you have to step outside of your comfort zone in the bedroom. No excuses. Stop having sex in the same spot, at the same time, in the same position! I don't care if you're wheelchair bound and require a human crane to get around the house. Use that crane to crash yourself down onto your husband waiting unexpectedly below!

Adding adventure into your sex life solves many typical relationship issues. An exciting sex life leads to appreciation, humor, loyalty, and so much more. When you have more passionate sex, every area of growth in your relationship is emphasized. Imagine how easy it will be to visualize what you are thankful for in your relationship after you've had a good shag in the woods. You'll appreciate how adventurous they are. You'll appreciate how good they look. You'll feel like your relationship has been renewed. Quality sex is necessary.

The creative options for enhancing your love life are endless! Don't let your fear of change get in the way. If you want to have the sex life you deserve, start thinking outside of the box. Come up with some unique ideas and discuss with your partner. Surprises can be romantic, but surprising your lover with kinky ropes and chains is probably not the best first step. Perhaps they have always wanted to try something wild or have a secret sexual bucket list they've never revealed to you. You'll never know until you take the (possibly uncomfortable) action and talk to them about their ambitions! Just like you shared your realistic expectations with each other; share your realistic sexual expectations with each other. This can be an uncomfortable subject, but by being direct with your partner you are one step closer to resolving your bedroom woes.

Once you have discussed some sensitive subjects with your lover, hopefully you will have a clearer understanding of their desires. Maybe they are completely satisfied with the way things are going and bringing home a XXX movie would terrify them. But that doesn't mean you can't spice things up. Maybe everything else in the bedroom stays the same, but you can take an extra romantic step that you hadn't considered. By simply making some chocolate covered strawberries or playing their favorite record, you can add an element of depth to your typical intimacy. However small your action is, I challenge you to implement at least one new idea into your bedroom life. Take action today to reinvigorate your intimacy and show your partner just how sexy you can be.

Consider resources such as kama sutra guides or a sex therapist. I know studying some new moves or learning from a professional isn't *sexy*. But, taking the initiative to explore avenues you haven't considered will lead to lasting excitement for you and your partner. Learning new techniques and exploring other bedroom options can be a useful strategy when trying to heal or reinvigorate your relationship. Worst case scenario, you try a bunch of new things only to realize that what you had going was already exciting enough. With the courage of exploration, you will have a better understanding of how to keep the fire in your relationship burning brightly.

Long distance intimacy

No matter which phase of love life you're in, distance in a relationship is bound to be a reality for you at some point. Distance between partners can be a major source of conflict in a relationship. But it doesn't have to be. Since you've made it this far, you already know that many of the principles presented in this book readily apply to a long-distance relationship. If you are practicing gratefulness for your partner, speaking their love language (physical touch is temporarily exempt), and encouraging their passions, love from afar will be a lot less painful.

My experience with distance love occurred while dating a marine. Our relationship was based on lustful desire and other unhealthy lifestyles. Both of us were in the relationship for the wrong reasons. We were having fun and it seemed like everything was getting along just fine. Little did we know, the upcoming distance in our relationship was about to expose just how flimsy our relationship was.

We were dating for a year before she was shipped off to boot camp. She had decided to join the marines before we had met, and I selfishly wanted her to abandon the plan. I believed my motives were pure; I was trying to manipulate her into staying because I felt that I needed her. Jealousy (visions of buff marines swooning her) and rage ("how dare she abandon me!") occupied my headspace. I selfishly used every tactic I could think of to try and sway her decision. I had successfully convinced myself that I was the victim and that she was the tormentor. I couldn't see it at the time, but I was lying to both of us. It was all about what I needed and I wasn't being considerate of her dreams.

Our superficial relationship was propped up almost entirely by sex and quickly lost its artificial support once she departed. We maintained a snail-mail correspondence for the three months apart while I continued to dwell in the victim mindset. Instead of being encouraging, appreciative, and a source of light in her life, I selfishly plodded onward in my attempts to manipulate her out of the dream. I'll spare you the rest of the heart-breaking details but as expected, the relationship ended during her first deployment following boot-camp.

In this case, distance was useful in exposing the inherent foundational weakness of my relationship. If you apply the principles outlined in this book, such as owning responsibility for your own happiness, practicing gratitude, self-awareness, and focusing on passions rather than how your partner can serve you, I believe that distance will create renewed closeness with your partner. Distance will become a non-issue when both of you understand these principles. Obviously, the one caveat to distance enhancing a relationship can be the lack of physical intimacy. It is necessary in a relationship, so having a concrete plan to reunite with each other should be defined. Until then, here are some ideas for keeping your relationship intact and your partner just as dedicated as you are.

Outside of physical intimacy, which love languages speak to their heart? If their primary love language is physical touch, this can be a challenge, but double down on other areas of love that are impactful for them. Your words of affirmation will become more meaningful. Your acts of service will become more apparent when they feel comforted knowing the house is taken care of. Your gifts will be prized and take on new meaning as the distance makes them realize how much they miss you. Use your imagination and utilize this time apart to show them that despite the distance you will always be there for them.

Although it may not seem like it after your first week apart, distance can have a profoundly positive influence in your relationship. Perhaps your relationship was too heavily centered around physical intimacy and the distance enhanced your listening and communication skills. Maybe the space provided you with the time you needed to find the motivation for organizing the garage. Instead of looking at the separation with despair, use this time to your advantage. By finding ways to connect with your partner from a distance, you will feel renewed appreciation for each other when you are finally together again.

Here are some solutions while separated to get your creative juices flowing:

- Create a photo diary of your favorite memories together and hide it in their suitcase or send it off to their hotel (Shutterfly.com provides an easy and affordable album service.)
- Send a handwritten love letter sealed with your perfume/cologne (Include photo of you and the dog!)
- Get out that lingerie/man thong and do some dirty dancing via webcam (or just call them for a

chat, chances are good you'll be talking more since they're gone!)

- Send them flowers (or their favorite 6-pack of beer via DoorDash/Instacart)
- Film and send a video of you conquering the one chore you've been putting off (use their most hated chore for maximum effect)

It's not rocket science, but a little extra shared compassion goes a long way. Spending five minutes on a video-chat to brighten their day is simple and will make the distance apart less painful. The rest of the day is yours! No nagging partner and unlimited couch time!   But seriously, alone time is vital. Embrace the calm and quiet home. Remember, they probably want some peace and quiet too, so limiting the communication might be a good idea if you usually spend every waking moment together and are always in contact.

Continue practicing thankfulness for everything that you have. Loneliness cannot exist when you keep your attention focused on the wonderful life you currently have. Instead of thinking, "I can't stand being alone," think about what you can be doing to better yourself. When your partner finally makes it home, they'll be met with a better you, reinforcing all of the reasons they already love you.

There are other advantages to learning how to love from a distance. Occasional separation from your loved one will uncover truths about your relationship that may have been forgotten. As I write, it's day one of five in my temporary bachelor pad. My love has gone down to visit with her sister for the week. Win-win for both of us. She gets a few days off of work, and gets to hang-out with her best-friend/sister; I get to enjoy quiet time, hikes with my dog, and am reminded of the many reasons why I love my lady.

The glaring truths about our relationship are made evident during these times apart, and we always grow closer together after these little breaks. I like to think of mini-solo trips as recalibration points in our relationship. After years together, the dreaded relationship routines attempt to creep onto the scene. I resist that creep constantly, and times apart supply an additional tool for supporting the exciting and fresh relationship I desire.

On the contrary, the truth-exposing nature of distance can have a detrimental effect on a relationship. If you're a victim in your relationship (physical or emotional abuse) and find a major sense of relief when you are separated, then this is an obvious indicator that your partner isn't right for you. Refer back to the section on having courage and removing yourself from toxic influences if distance has revealed that your relationship is beyond repair.

Breaking up is hard to do

Let go, or be dragged. -Zen Proverb

There's no simple solution to ending a relationship that is beyond repair. I want to emphasize the importance of doing everything within your power to heal and improve your relationship before giving up too quickly. If you feel like you've exhausted all of your options and all of your relationship improvement efforts have been in vain then the next unfortunate step is to jump-ship. Only you can decide if this drastic step is appropriate. While it is ultimately up to you to decide, I challenge you to refer back to the list of gratitudes that you created earlier. Hold yourself accountable and accurately gauge if you have truly given it your all. Did you start making some changes for the better or did you gradually regress to your old patterns that led to the initial problems?

Our natural instincts incline us to hyper-focus on the issues rather than re-living the beautiful moments together. Despite your best efforts to retain a fulfilling relationship, you are met with separation and seeming disaster. Don't let yourself become a victim in this scenario. The gratitude you have learned to practice while with your partner is equally relevant in a break-up situation. Instead of allowing anger to rule your head-space, reflect on all of the joyful moments that taught you how to open your heart to another.

Oftentimes, you will be faced with a one-sided decision to separate. You may be blind-sided by your partner, naively thinking that your deep-love for them was reciprocated. If you have faced a scenario like this, it can often leave you wondering where you went wrong.

It isn't always up to you. Despite your best efforts to keep your relationship afloat, there will be times when your efforts fall upon deaf ears. Do not despair, rather, try to understand why the relationship didn't work out and double-down on self-healing and care. If you know you have given your all to your partner, the failure of that relationship is likely a reflection of their own internal discontent.

Time spent with another person in harmony and passion is never wasted, even if it didn't turn out the way you had hoped. Each and every one of my failed relationships has helped to strengthen my resolve, increase my patience, and learn to transform frustrations into inner-calmness. Once you have learned to live a life with less attachment to external influences, your internal landscape will take on a resilience that can weather any emotional storm.

The pain of separation will be very real. You have a choice to reside with that pain, or you can harness that powerful emotion to propel you forward into a stronger and more contented you. Once you truly love yourself and understand your intrinsic value, it's their loss if they're unable to recognize those values. At the end of the day, you can always count on yourself.

It's never too late to start again

Getting back out there and finding love again can seem like a terrifying prospect. With a simple shift in your methodology, you'll find that the process can happen much more naturally than you'd expect. My two suggestions to get you started: Focus on your passions and you'll come across someone that enjoys similar activities and give online dating a chance.

While factoring a new relationship into your life that's rooted in shared passions, you'll be primed for success. The goal here is to maximize your chance of success while minimizing time spent on fruitless dating. If you have a string of failed relationships littering your past, then you already know how much time you've wasted on people that never came close to aligning with your basic criteria.

Oftentimes, fruitless dating comes from having a short-term outlook that is based on unrealistic expectations or personal emotional deficits. For example, a week after one of my break-ups, I met a girl at one of the local bars. The entire foundation of that relationship started on rocky ground. We were both drunk, we didn't know anything about each other's long term plans or passions, and launched into physical intimacy mindlessly. Subconsciously, my unrealistic expectation was that this person was somehow magically going to mesh well with my life. I was focused on the superficial aspects and the temporary broken-heart band-aide she provided instead of taking the time to lay a healthy groundwork.

I know this is cliche, but becoming friends with someone you plan on dating is a great idea and will prevent a failed scenario like this. It's important that you understand the person under the hood before you get tied up in romance. Obviously there are exceptions, but why take unnecessary risk when finding an ideal match is so important.

The problem is that we choose our relationships with passion, not logic. Deciding whom we are going to spend our precious time with shouldn't be a snap decision based on a fleeting feeling while blinded by lust. Again, there are exceptions, but wouldn't you rather take the cautious approach when investing (potentially) the rest of your life?

Hopefully you can agree and will opt for a more logical dating route instead. The online dating route. Yes, I'm a hypocrite for dissing the tech-revolution earlier because I failed to mention that I met my lovely lady through an online dating site. There are significant advantages when utilizing technology for discovering romance. The world of dating will never be the same again, for better and for worse. Fortunately, I was lucky enough to come across an amazing woman that aligned with many of my relationship criteria and realistic expectations.

What eventually opened my heart up to the idea of online dating was a lesson taught to us in my 9th grade biology class. I'll never forget the phenomenal scientific analogy when discussing his views on dating: Do the proteins in our body find the compatible cells randomly? No, they are targeted to a particular cell because they contain a specific amino acid sequence that causes them to bind to the appropriate receptors. This analogy can be applied to our dating life. What are the chances that we randomly stumble upon someone that we are highly compatible with in our day to day lives? While it is possible, the odds aren't in our favor. Fortunately, by utilizing a dating service or by putting ourselves in the right passion filled activities, we can automatically eliminate many candidates that don't synthesize with our passions and goals. Do anything you can to increase your odds of success, even if that means listening to my high school teacher's advice.

Sadly, many of these dating apps have become outlets for temporary pleasure and vanity. Despite the glaring flaws, online opportunities have the potential to get your relationship started on a solid foundation. The proteins have **specific** chains of amino acids for a reason. You need to be **specific** when developing a framework of dating criteria.

Think about the passions and realistic expectations you uncovered earlier. I recommend creating a list with your most important relationship goals, and rate these goals from highest priority to lowest. If your criteria of aspirations for a relationship are too strict, then you may be limited on the prospects you come across. Some flexibility is necessary, but be sure to have items that you are unwilling to compromise on.

You'll be amazed to see how many people on the dating platforms have similar aspirations. If you ever thought, "I'm just bad at relationships," then you'll gladly learn that with the appropriate criteria in place, someone that is highly compatible to you is readily available. There are plenty of fish in the sea, and that's why I recommend the free to use site PlentyOfFish.Com or the less free- MeetMindful.Com. There are too many useful apps and sites to list here, but any of them will do if you stick to your pre-defined relationship guidelines.

The virtual dating life isn't for everyone. If you have successfully identified passions that bring you to life, love may be right under your nose. Refer back to your list of passions and decide if anything on your list could guide you towards a potential date. When you are engaged in the activities you love, the people sharing in that passion will be drawn to you. Immerse yourself in those passions. Developing a deep connection with someone that is equally alive in their passion will increase your odds of compatibility and shared joy in life.

Be courageous. All of the self-growth you've cultivated is only the start. Use your newfound love-skills and start branching out. If you're in a billiards club, take the next step and actually *talk* to that cute guy you've been eyeing across the table. If you love to read, join a book club. Whatever you're passionate about, figure out a way to share it with others. All of your dreams of finding love can only come true if you're willing to take the action required. When you become steadfast in your goals and passions, confidence will replace doubt. This will not happen over-night, but as your self-worth increases, so will your ability to recognize the opportunities available to you.

Falling in love with a friend is cliche, but thanks to shared passions, friendships often blossom into lasting love. Instead of trapping yourself in *the friend zone*, ask yourself: Are any of your current friends potentially compatible with you? Think back to the realistic expectations from earlier. If they check all of your boxes, what are you waiting for?

Be patient. Perhaps the timing isn't quite right. You've found the person of your dreams, but maybe they are already in a relationship. It shouldn't matter, because if you continue practicing an attitude of self-appreciation and contentment with your own life, there's no reason to rush. You are happy with yourself, remember? Love is just the frosting on life's cake. Even if you have flourished into the person you would want to spend time with, love isn't guaranteed. Continue growing and exploring things that bring you joy.

If you are living to your fullest potential while keeping an open heart and mind, love will find you. No matter how tempting random flings may seem, resist those temporary trappings. Remain resolute in your non-compromising criteria of realistic expectations. Seriously, don't cheat yourself. Even if it takes years to find someone that you are compatible with, don't lose sight of your end goal. Continue growing into the person you want to be. As your passions evolve over the years, so will your aspirations in love. If you settle for a mediocre love from the beginning, that's what you'll end up with. Don't settle.

Final thoughts and encouragement

When faced with the complexities of love, you're destined to face a number of hurdles along your journey. There will always be new reasons why something doesn't go the way you had planned. Oftentimes, the lowest points in your love journey may leave you feeling hopeless. It is okay if you feel defeated at times, but refuse to let these temporary situations define your long term aspirations. Hopefully you will adopt some of the principles throughout this book and will be able to continue along your path with a renewed sense of awareness and hope.

Have you come up with some realistic additions to your love arsenal? It is my greatest wish that you come to find lasting love. For all the hopeless romantics, day dreamers, and gentle souls that feel lost in this dark world, never give up on your love goals. Hold the reason for desiring a healthy love life in the foreground of your mind and keep your eyes open for the ever-available opportunities that are in alignment with your dreams.

As you progress through your love journey, I challenge you to keep a catalogue of your experiences. I want you to maintain a record of what works, what doesn't work, and where you feel that improvement is needed. I want to emphasize the earlier point of maintenance of your love skills. Learning to be consistent and continually challenging yourself to grow will be a lifelong pursuit with your newfound love strategies. When you feel that the romance is fading, or you are being less than attentive, get to the root of these issues quickly. When you feel that you are straying from your long-term love aspirations, it is important that you hold yourself accountable. Continue to practice intentional love with consistent action. You must hold yourself to a high standard if you hope to maintain the love you have been blessed with.

In a recent discussion I shared with my love, we were contemplating the intricacies of what drives our motivations in life. The only constant when striving towards our aspirations is a constant fluctuation of internal and external motivating factors. We unanimously agreed that while both the internal and external contributing factors were relevant, the internal drivers have a more lasting impact.

As the external reason for doing anything in life begins to fade, we must dwell on the internal reasoning for accomplishing anything that demands focused effort. Reflect back on your primary reasons for what you hope to achieve in love. These internal drivers can sustain you throughout your greatest difficulties. If you're able to notice the simple pleasures along the way, that's just an added bonus.

As our discussion drifted along, we both smiled at each other reassuringly. Sharing in the knowledge that despite whatever the world had in store for us, our intrinsic motivators to continue loving each other would prevail. We have found an unconditional love that resides deep within our hearts that will last into our later years. Perhaps I am naive, perhaps I am an eternal optimist, or perhaps I have finally failed enough times. I have learned to gratefully accept the ebb and flow of love without judgement or expectation.

You deserve a love worth fighting for.

Are you ready to fight for love?

A special thanks to my family and friends for being wonderful examples of what it means to love unconditionally.

References:

The 5 Love Languages - Gary D. Chapman

Joe Rogan Motivational Speech:
https://youtu.be/SZEo1KFjTn4

A New Earth - Eckhart Tolle

The Science of Getting Rich – Wallace D. Wattles

The Subtle Art of Not Giving a F*ck – Mark Manson

A Liberated Mind - Steven C. Hayes

The Power of Habit - Charles Duhigg

The 4 Hour Work-Week - Timothy Ferris

Rich Dad, Poor Dad - Robert Kiyosaki

www.ingramcontent.com/pod-product-compliance
Lightning Source LLC
Chambersburg PA
CBHW061338250726
48657CB00004B/1219